Speech Therapy Aphasia Rehabilitation *STAR*

Workbook III

Naming and Describing

Amanda Anderson M.S. CCC-SLP

Cover Photo: NGC 6946 Galaxy via: NASA[i]

Table of Contents

DEDICATION

Dedicated to David Dow and Aphasia Recovery Connection, emulating the finest qualities of strength and perseverance. I am fortunate to have worked with you. Your determination and energy have helped shape me into the therapist I am today.

Forward

by: Dr. Jodi Dodds, Vascular Neurologist

Language and communication enable us to function as a society. We exchange information with our families, our neighbors, our colleagues, those with whom we are involved in transactions. We find the right things to say, and when there is nothing that can be said, we listen empathetically in understanding of what others convey to us in conversation. We laugh at the humor in jokes, and we feel angry when hurtful words come our way. Spoken and comprehended language enhances what we feel hundreds of times each day.

When I first began treating stroke patients as a vascular neurologist, I thought the greatest challenges I would face would involve physical disabilities: weakness in an arm or a leg, or difficulties people would face with balance when ambulating. What I quickly learned was that aphasia, or disruptions in expressed or interpreted language, can be just as disabling as a severe physical limitation. Patients with aphasia have shared similar stories with me. These are stories of efforts to formulate comments during a family dinner discussion, only to find that once the language is processed and ready to be spoken, the conversation has moved on to a different topic. Patients claim they experience complex thoughts and ideas, but find frustration when their words fail them. I have heard tales from English teachers who have read one book each week for 30 years, only to find that after their strokes it may take months to complete a book, and retaining what they have read may require reading and rereading the same paragraphs three or four times.

One of the valuable evidence-based resources for patients struggling with aphasia is speech therapy as part of their rehabilitation plan. If they quality with their particular medical insurance plan, in particular if an accompanying physical deficit is also present after a brain injury, a patient with aphasia may start his or her rehabilitation journey at an acute rehabilitation facility with daily therapy in an attempt to optimize early recovery. After discharging from acute rehabilitation, patients will then usually undergo speech therapy either at home or in an outpatient clinic, although less frequently (perhaps 2-3 times each week). Once a patient is deemed to have "plateaued," meaning the patient is no longer demonstrating objective, measurable progress, he or she is often discharged from speech therapy as this may no longer be covered under the patient's medical insurance. Another common scenario is that a patient may receive a specified number of speech therapy visits under a particular health plan, and once these are exhausted, formal speech therapy stops.

My advice to patients in these scenarios who felt they could still make further progress and were motivated to continue working independently to rehabilitate themselves used to be fairly limited. I would advise them to read as much as possible, and to attempt to discuss what they were reading with friends or family members. Read the newspaper, I would recommend, circle words that are unfamiliar, and ask a designated family member each day what they are, or try to utilize a dictionary. Engage in conversation with someone who is calm and patient, and continue to practice regular dialogue. Babies do not learn to speak and comprehend language overnight, but over years, and recovering from aphasia following a significant brain injury usually does not happen overnight either.

I first met Amanda Anderson, SLP, in 2011. She often worked with stroke patients in her career as a speech language pathologist, and had the same feelings of concern for patients who were discharged from speech therapy but were still motivated to progress further with language recovery. In 2013, she brought a copy of her first aphasia workbook, *Speech Therapy Aphasia Rehabilitation Workbook: Expressive and Written Language*, to the neurology clinic where I see patients, and I was quickly impressed. I showed the book to several patients, who purchased it and started working through the exercises. They returned for follow up visits and wanted to know if there was a second volume available. Their families commented that the book motivated them to continue with engagement in their own recoveries. I am thrilled to finally have a useful, affordable option to offer patients with aphasia who want to do more.

Ms. Anderson has now completed a third volume, *Speech Therapy Aphasia Rehabilitation *STAR* Workbook III: Expressive Language*, focusing largely on receptive expressive language deficits, and opening independent language rehabilitation to a new group of patients afflicted with aphasia.

I am personally grateful for the opportunity to offer my patients an additional tool in their aphasia recovery journey, and recommend both of these workbooks to any physician or medical provider treating stroke patients or populations of patients who have sustained brain injury with residual aphasia.

Jodi A. Dodds, MD
Vascular Neurologist
Charlotte, NC

Introduction

This workbook was created for people with aphasia to use with their speech therapist or with a caregiver at home. Unfortunately, insurance often doesn't cover speech therapy long enough to regain prior communication levels. This workbook is meant to serve as a supplement to therapy or to guide family through therapy to improve expressive language.

The key to successful aphasia speech therapy is to build new neurological pathways. After a stroke resulting in aphasia, the words and knowledge haven't been forgotten. The language center of the brain (Broca's area) is typically in the left hemisphere. Aphasia is a result of damage to this area of the brain from a stroke either caused by lack of oxygen (ischemic stroke) or bleeding in the brain (hemorrhagic stroke).

Speech therapy works by recruiting undamaged areas of the brain to help retrieve appropriate words during expressive communication. A person with aphasia can use gestures, writing, sounds, music, rhythm and other descriptive terms to utilize other areas of the brain to improve expressive language.

Think of a stroke as a road block in the brain. The words are still there but the pathways to retrieve them have been damaged. The goal of therapy is to use other "roads" to retrieve the words. Music, rhythm, gestures, adjectives and adverbs help the brain find other routes to communicate. The brain is capable of creating new neurological pathways to work around damaged areas. Speech therapy helps create these pathways and this workbook is a helpful tool to improve communication skills after a stroke. Aphasia is not a memory disorder and using exercises with well know phrases, songs and sayings help utilize memory to increase the brain's ability to form "detours" around the "road block" to improve expressive language.

Frequent practice of these exercises increases the formation of new neurological pathways to improve communication. Try to use the exercises from this workbook daily. Repetition of successful language activities helps increase communication. If you get frustrated, take a break. Frustration is a natural part of aphasia therapy. Frustration can exacerbate word finding difficulties and it is especially important to learn to relax and not let frustration become a form of language blockage.

The most important thing for a family member or caregiver to remember is that true aphasia does not damage cognitive abilities. Remind your partner that you understand they know the answer and they are just having difficulty expressing it. The answers to the questions in the workbook are designed to be easy and they are not meant to question the patient's intelligence but rather to improve their ability to retrieve words. Aphasia is not a progressive disease. There is a strong potential for recovery of language skills with therapy, motivation and a lot of support.

How To Use This Workbook
For Family and Caregivers

This workbook can be used by your speech-language pathologist who will understand what types of cues you will need to improve your speech production. A speech therapist can use this book to structure your therapy to improve your expressive language.

This workbook is also designed to be used at home by the patient individually or with the help of a family member. The exercises are structured by difficulty level and each exercise is an opportunity to improve word retrieval skills. Everyone has experienced the feeling of having a word on the "tip of their tongue". Keep in mind, somebody with aphasia has this experience constantly and struggles to find the words they want to say even though they know what they want to say.

In the section for Functional Picture Naming, the objective is for the person with aphasia to name the item in the photograph. If they have trouble, use the carrier phrases below each picture. The questions below each photo are designed to help form new pathways to increase expressive language. Finding other ways to describe an item by function, or using a gesture, helps work around the area of the brain that was damaged. Try having your partner write the name of the picture. Depending on the type of stroke, writing can be just as difficult as speaking or it can be unaffected and a perfect mode of communication to help facilitate speech. If your partner is unable to name or answer any of the questions about the photo, write the name of the picture on an index card and place it below the picture. Have them read it with the picture. Practice reading the words with the pictures and gradually remove the written cue once they are able to read the name with the photograph on a consistent basis.

Safety Awareness Photographs: Aphasia does not impact intelligence but often stroke survivors have to adjust to new physical limitations. This section of photographs provide opportunities to improve safety awareness to prevent falls and practice how to ask for help with improve expressive language skills. The photographs are meant to initiate discussion about safety. In addition to answering the questions about the pictures, describe the details in the photo, describe personal obstacles related to the photograph and practice reviewing safety strategies. If the person with aphasia participates in physical therapy, this is a good opportunity to incorporate their safety goals and strategies into speech therapy. Have them write their safety goals down and practice reading them with you.

Sequences: Discuss the steps involved to complete the task. Describe each photograph in the sequence as completely as possible. Compare the task to how the person with aphasia does the task themselves. Use the photo sequences to launch into discussion about personal experience using gestures, descriptions and the photographs as cues to increase expressive language production. For a more challenging exercise, after the person with aphasia looks at the photo sequences have them describe the steps involved in completing the task without looking at the photographs. Every photograph provides an opportunity for the person with aphasia to increase use of descriptive language by describing all the details in the photo, discussing when the picture was taken, where it was and as a challenge why and how something is happening.

Describing compare contrast. This section contains different photographs of cakes and homes. Have the person with aphasia describe each photo with as much detail as possible. After they describe each photo, have them discuss which one they like the best. If they have a seen a similar object or which one they particularity dislike. As a challenge, have them discuss the similarities and differences between some of the objects in this section.

Descriptive Photographs: In addition to answering the questions about each photo, this section is designed to launch conversations about a variety of subjects. The goal for this exercise is to have your partner give as much detail about each photo as possible. Naming isn't the goal here. Try giving them the book without knowing the picture they are looking at. Encourage them to describe colors, people, time of year, location etc. Use the pictures to start conversations about places and personal experiences.

If you use the book in a group setting, have a person with aphasia describe a photograph to the group without directly naming it. It is similar to charades but talking is required in addition to gestures. The group should try to guess what the photograph is and each member of the group could try to draw a picture of what they think it looks like. The only rule is that the person who is describing can't just name the photograph. For example, for owl picture, the person with aphasia would say something like: "beak, big eyes, flies at night, smart, feathers, eats mice, makes pellets with bones, standing on one leg, on stump, swoop, brown, spotted, fluffy, talons, yellow eyes, etc."

Speech therapy for aphasia can be a long process. Remember that progress does happen. Patient motivation is a key factor for recovery. Warm up with activities from the book that are easy. Move on to more difficult sections but only for 10 to 15 minutes if they are frustrating for your partner. Cool down with activities that are easier. Frequent success and a lot of practice is the key to improving expressive language skills. Don't be afraid to ask friends and family for help. The opportunity to visit with friends can go a long way for a person with aphasia's rehabilitation. It is far better to speak all the time with multiple mistakes than to hardly speak at all with few mistakes. Consistent activity and opportunities to communicate help with recovery of expressive language function.

Naming

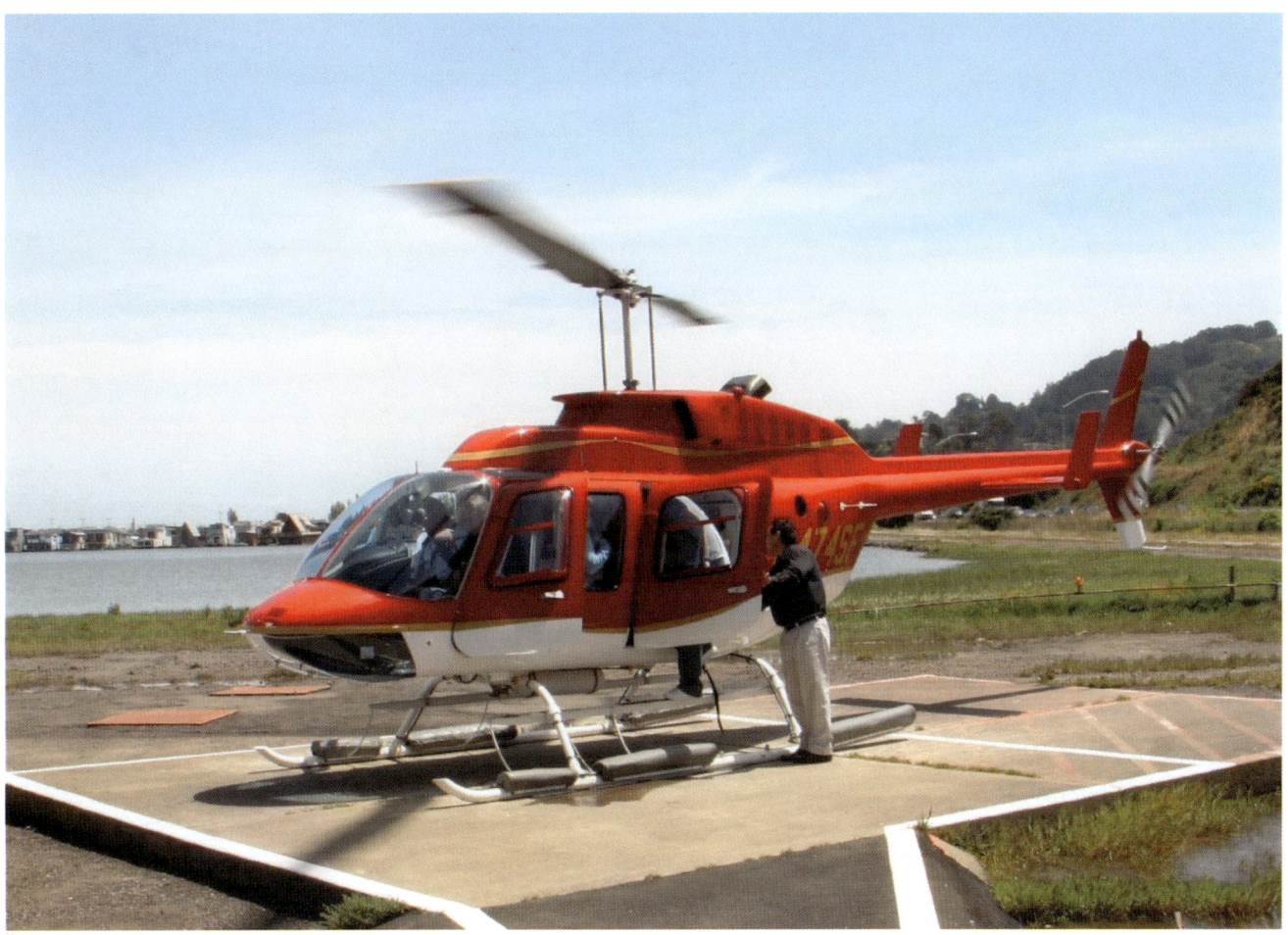

1. He was emergency airlifted to the hospital in a _____.

2. What does it do?

3. Who uses them?

4. How does it fly?

5. Make a gesture showing how it moves.

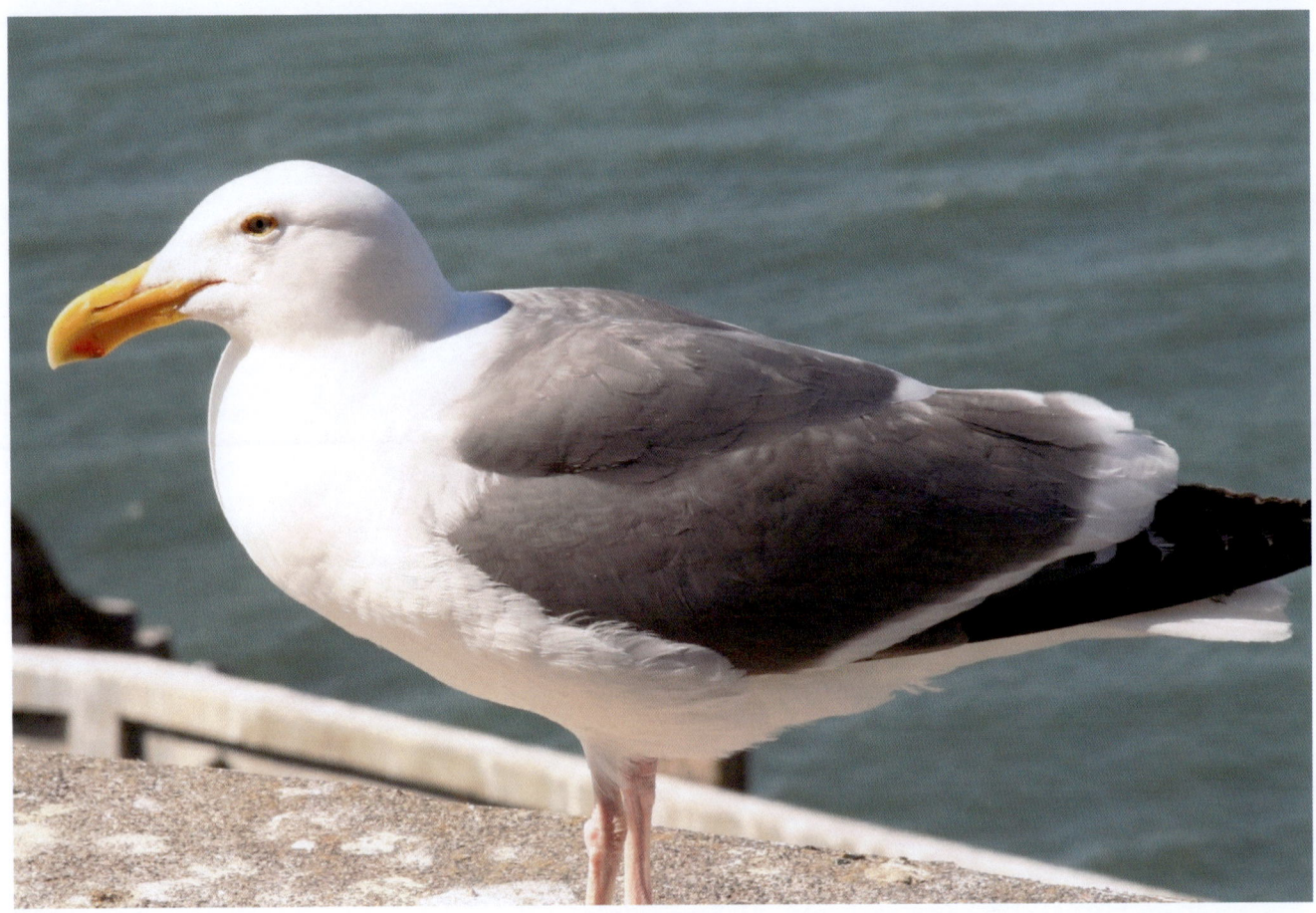

iii

1. Don't feed the _____.

2. Where do you find them?

3. What do they eat?

4. What sound do they make?

5. Make a gesture showing how it flies.

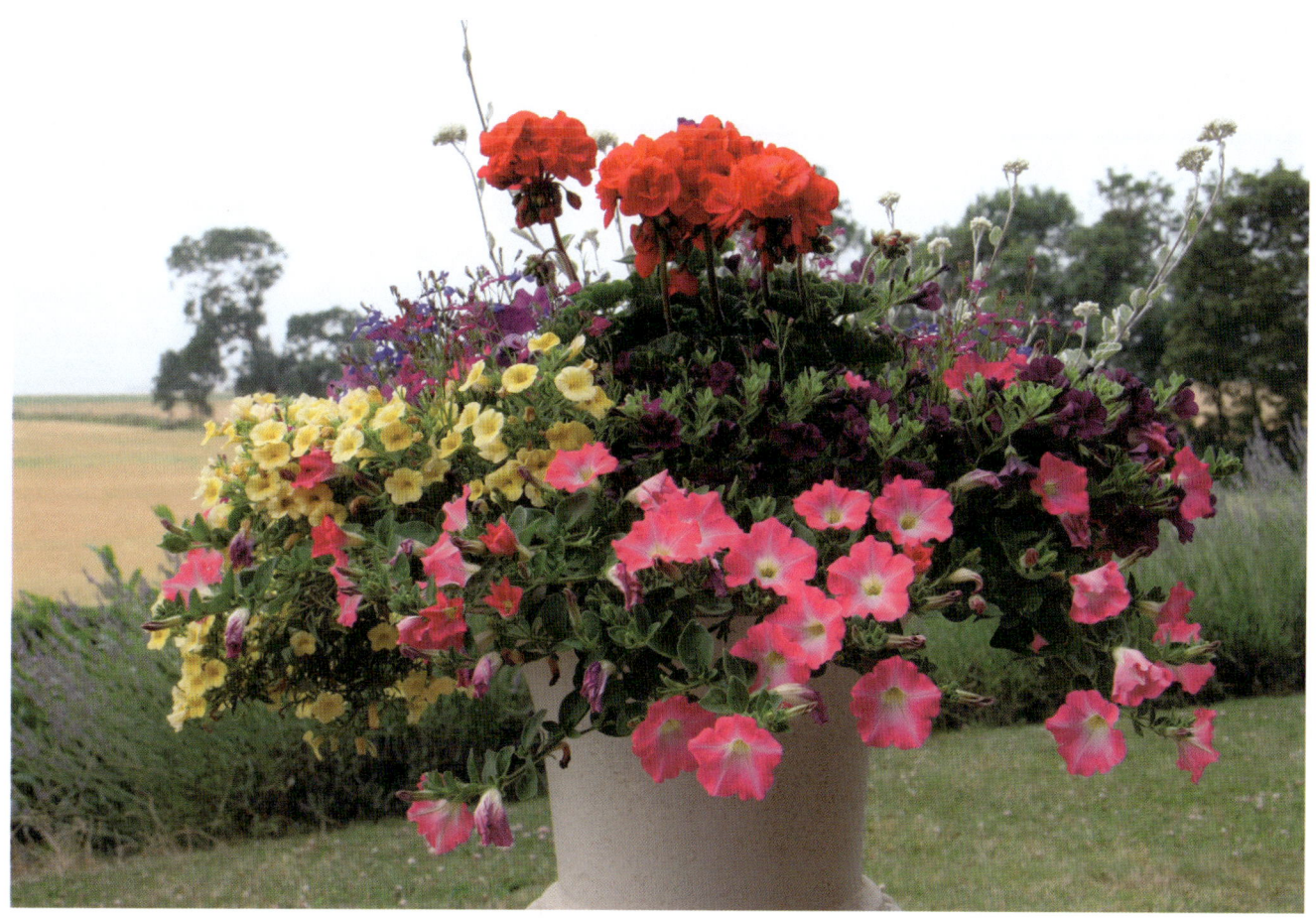

iv

1. Wow, what pretty _____.

2. What colors are they?

3. What are they growing out of?

4. When do they grow?

5. Pretend you are smelling them.

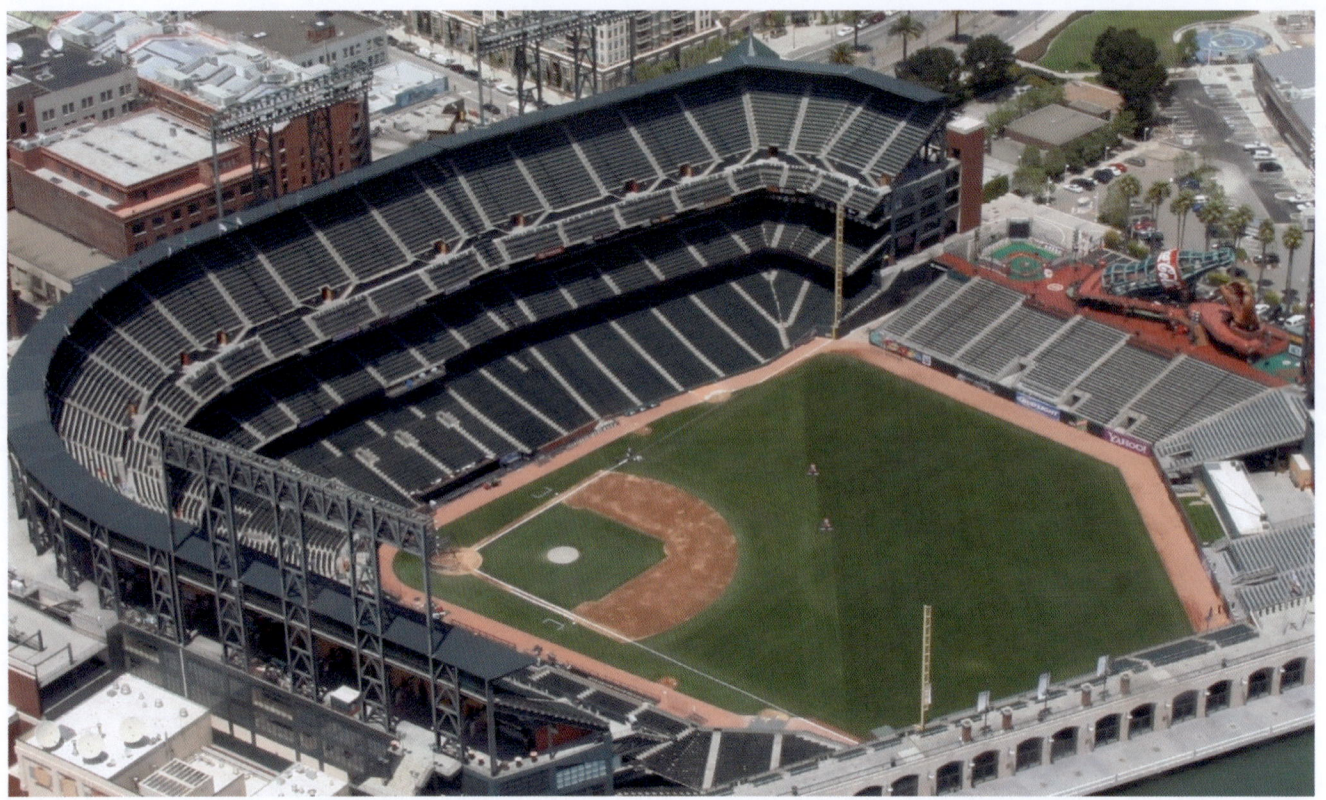

v

1. The blimp circled the baseball _____.

2. What is it for?

3. Who plays there?

4. What time of year do people go there?

5. Pretend you are up to bat.

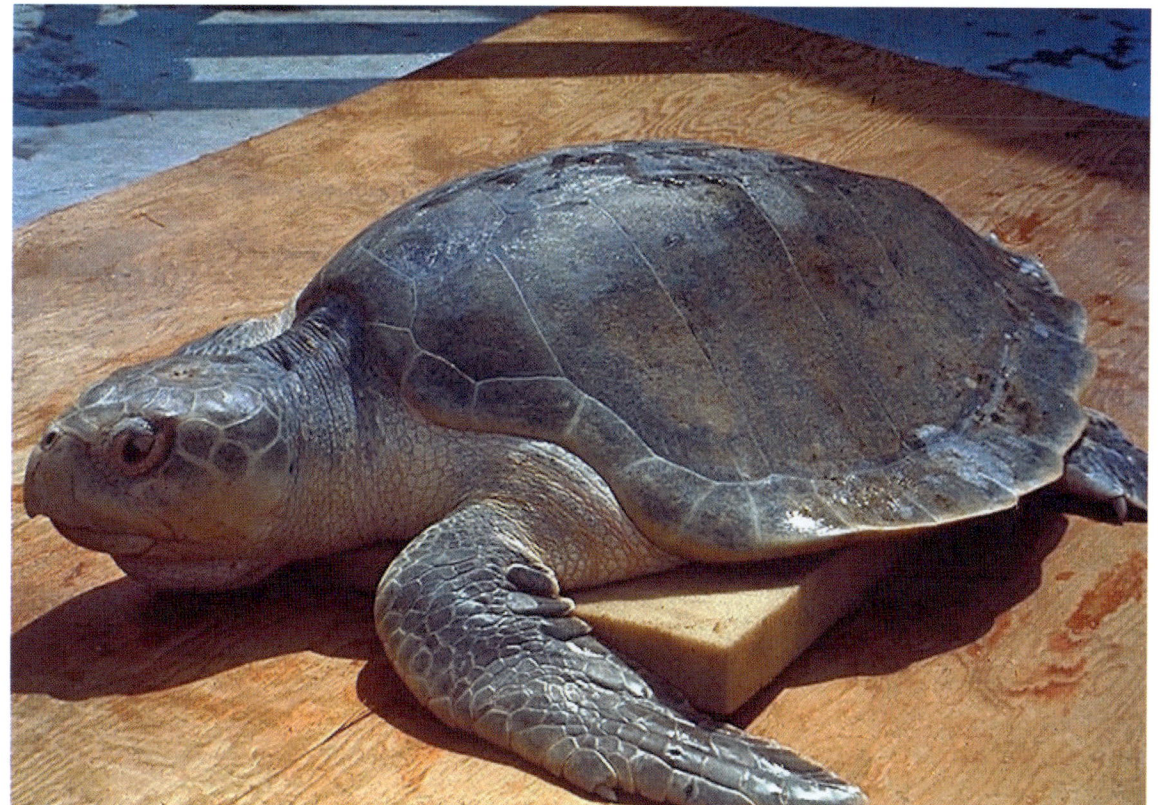

vi

1. When we were on vacation we saw a _____.

2. Where do they live?

3. Where do they lay their eggs?

4. How do they move?

5. Pretend to swim like one.

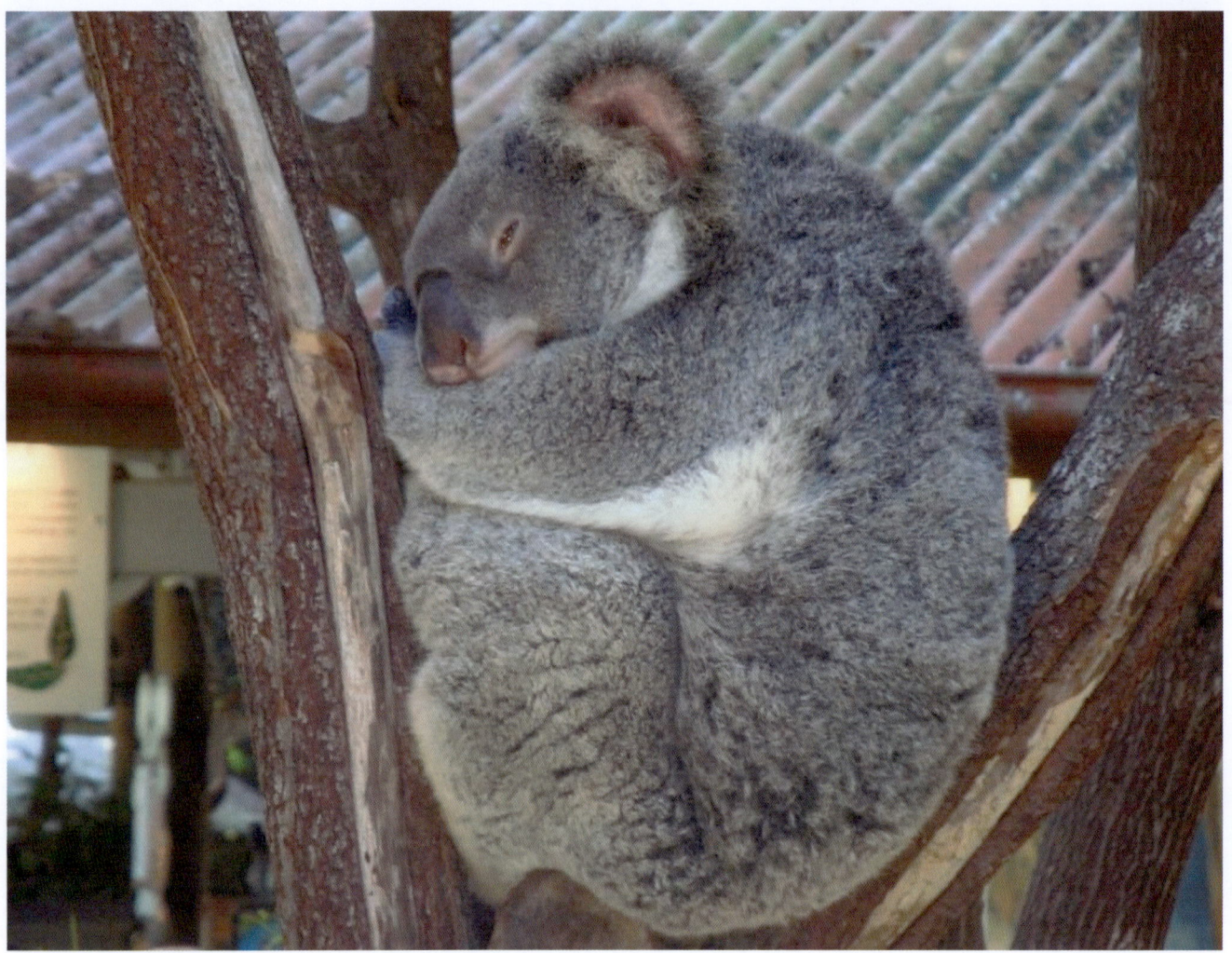

vii

1.   Look at that cute sleeping _____.

2.   What color is it?

3.   Where is it?

4.   What does it eat?

5.   Pretend you are sleeping too.

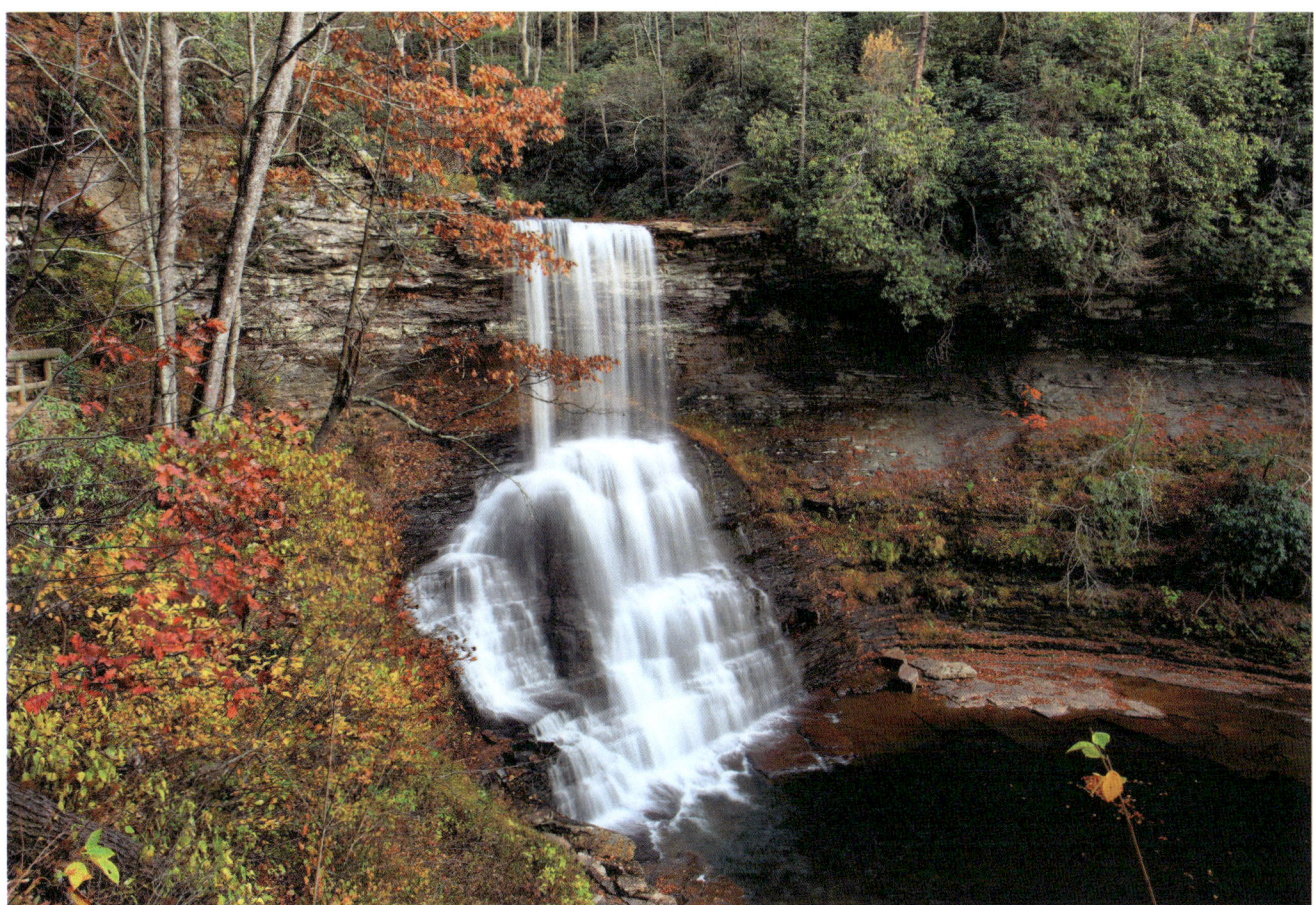

viii

1.   Look at the beautiful _____.

2.   Where do you find them?

3.   What are they made out of?

4.   Name a famous one.

5.   Make a gesture showing how they flow.

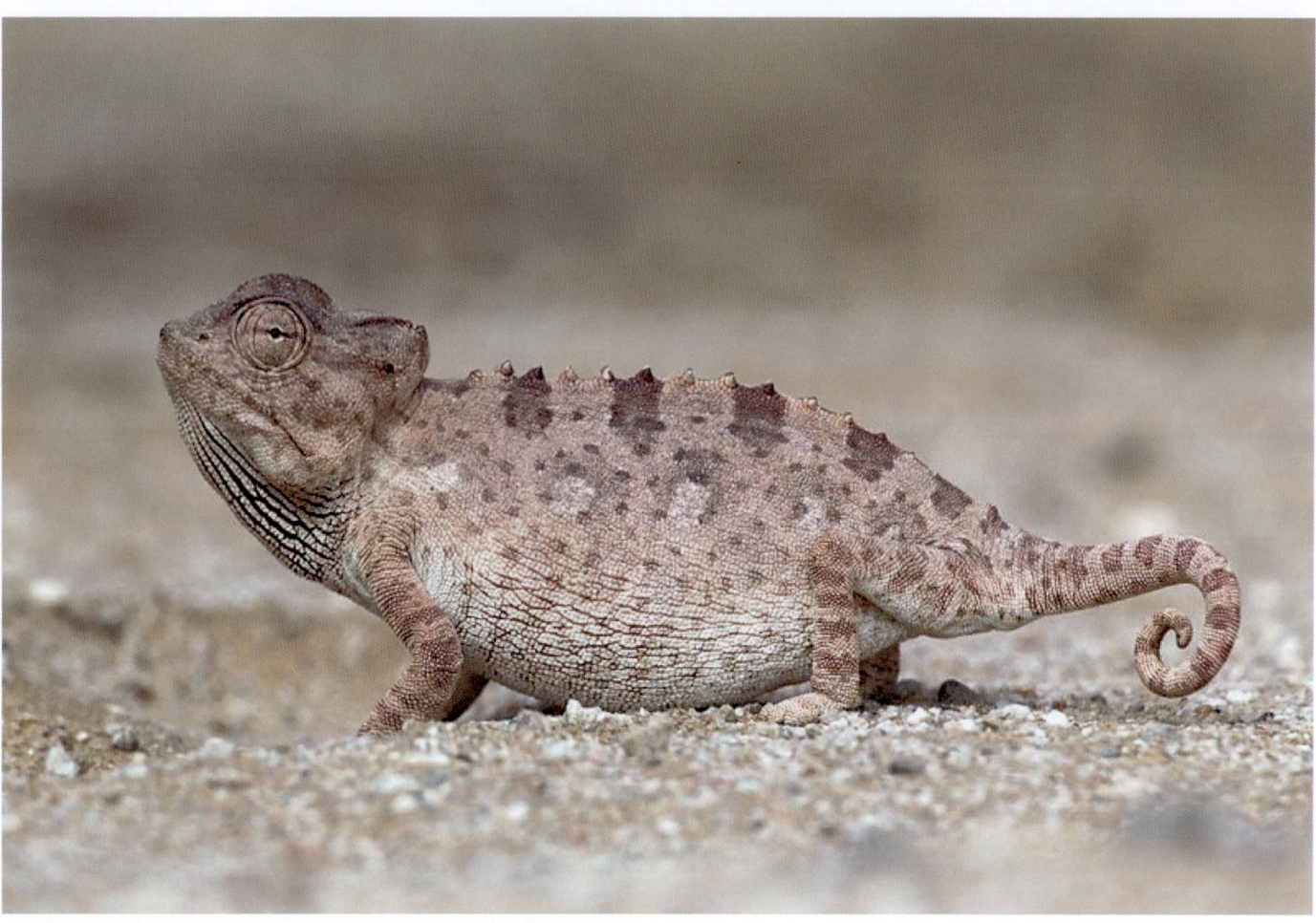

ix

1.   Look at the cute camouflaged _____.

2.   Where do you find them?

3.   What do they eat?

4.   What color is it?

5.   Pretend you have one on your arm.

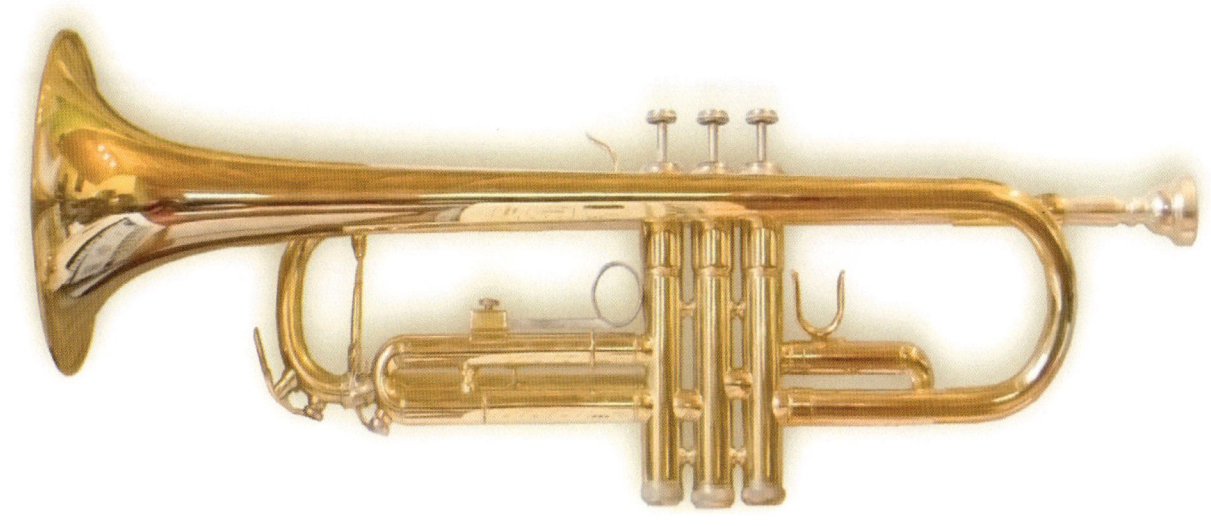

x

1. Dizzy Gillespie was famous for playing the _____.

2. Where would you see one?

3. What does it do?

4. Who uses them?

5. Pretend you are playing one.

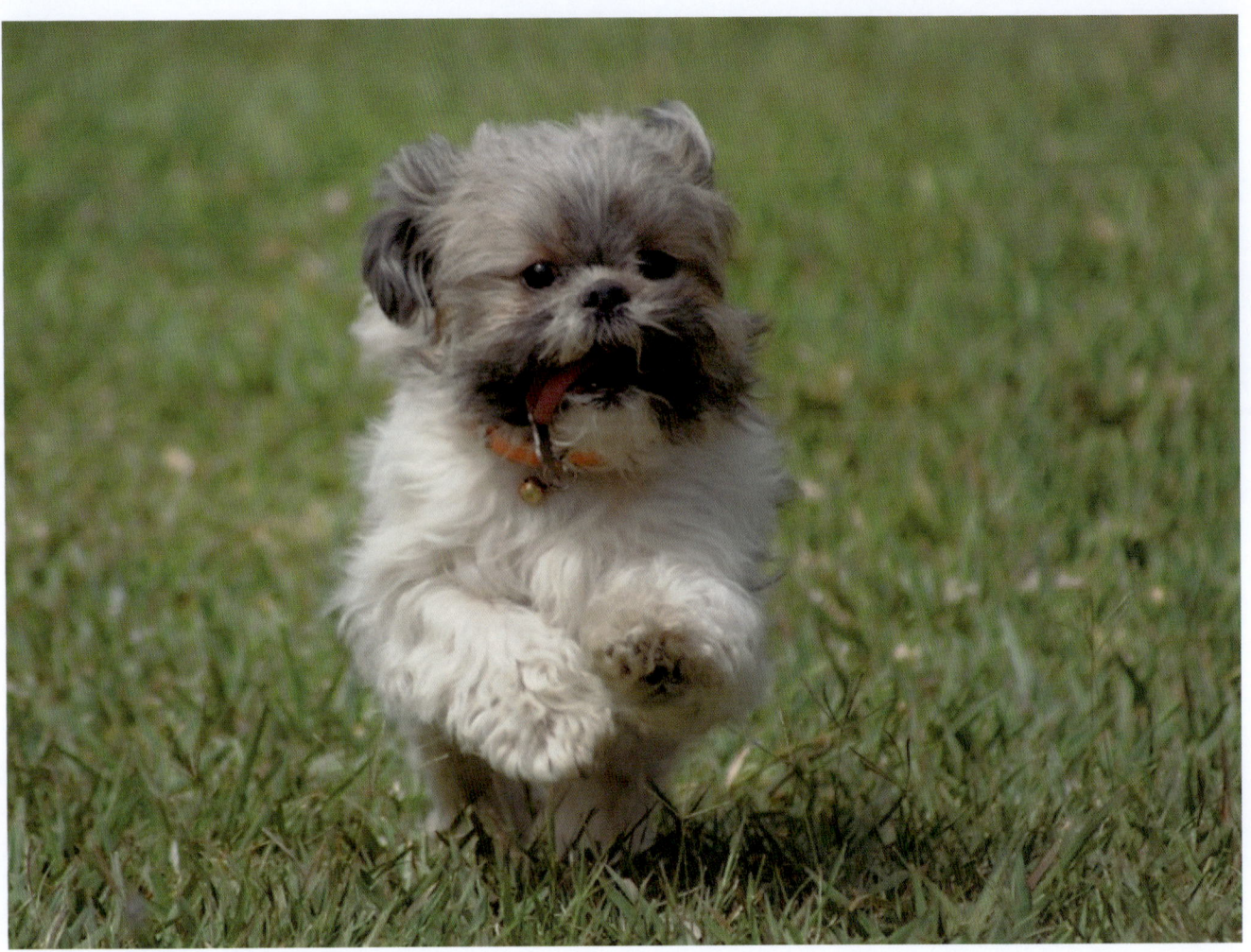

xi

1.   Would you like to pet my _____?

2.   How old do you think it is?

3.   Describe the puppy's hair?

4.   What is this puppy doing?

5.   What is your favorite dog breed?

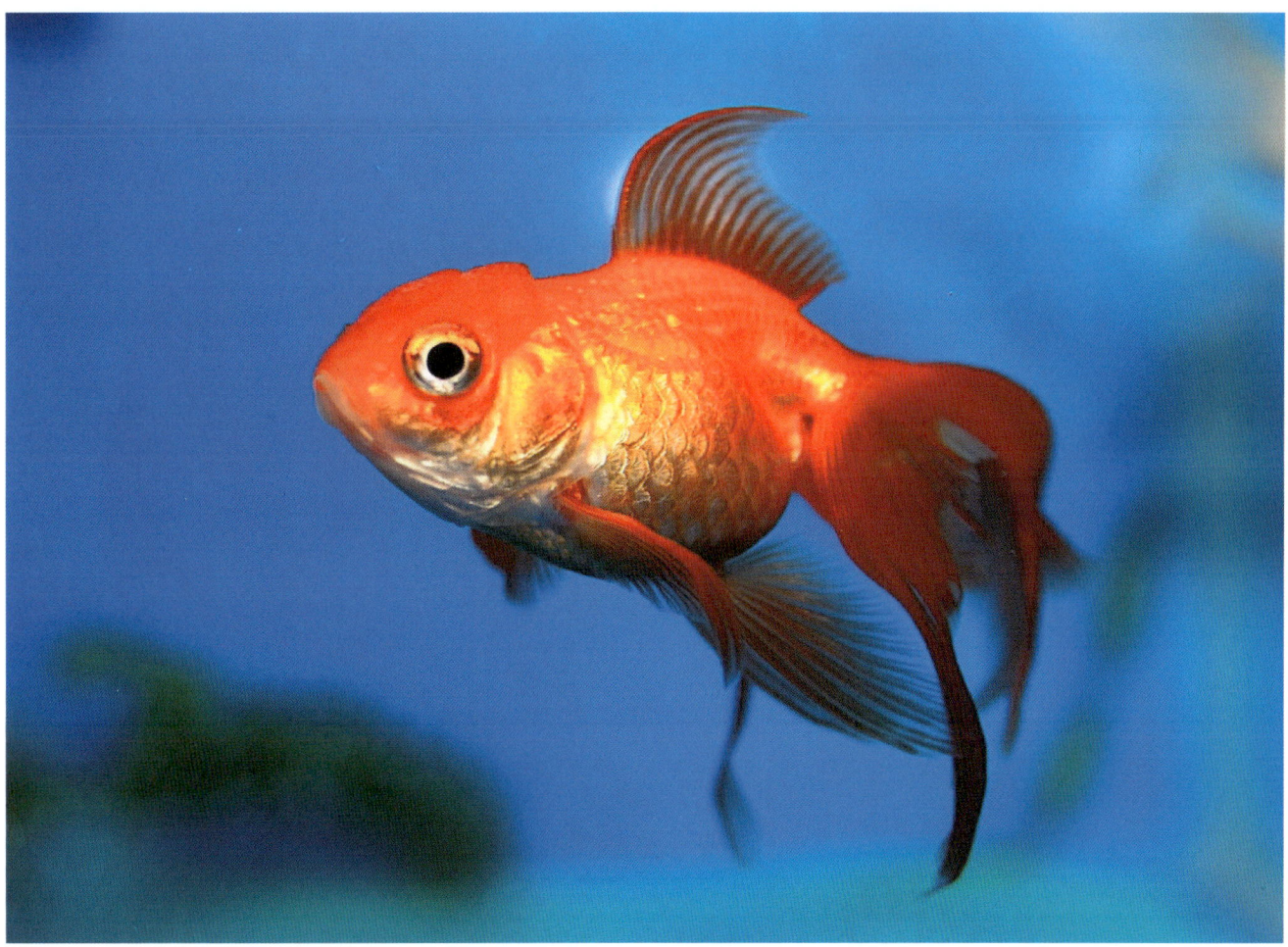

1.   Before I leave the house, I need to feed my gold_____.

2.   Where does it live?

3.   What does it eat?

4.   How does it move?

5.   Make a face like one.

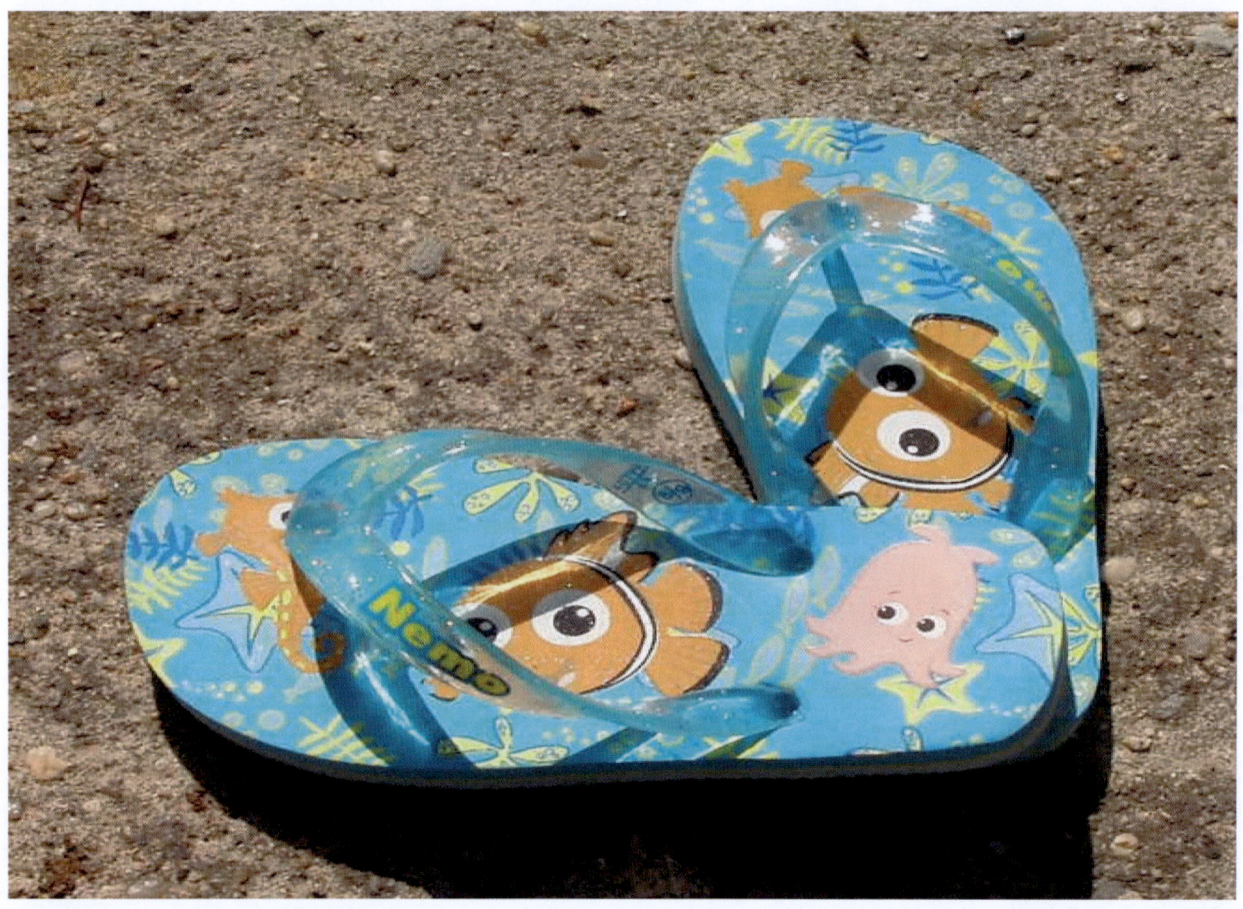

xiii

1.   Before I leave for the beach, I put on a pair of _____.

2.   Who would wear these?

3.   Where would you wear these?

4.   What time of year would you wear them?

5.   Make a sound mimicking how they sound when you walk in them.

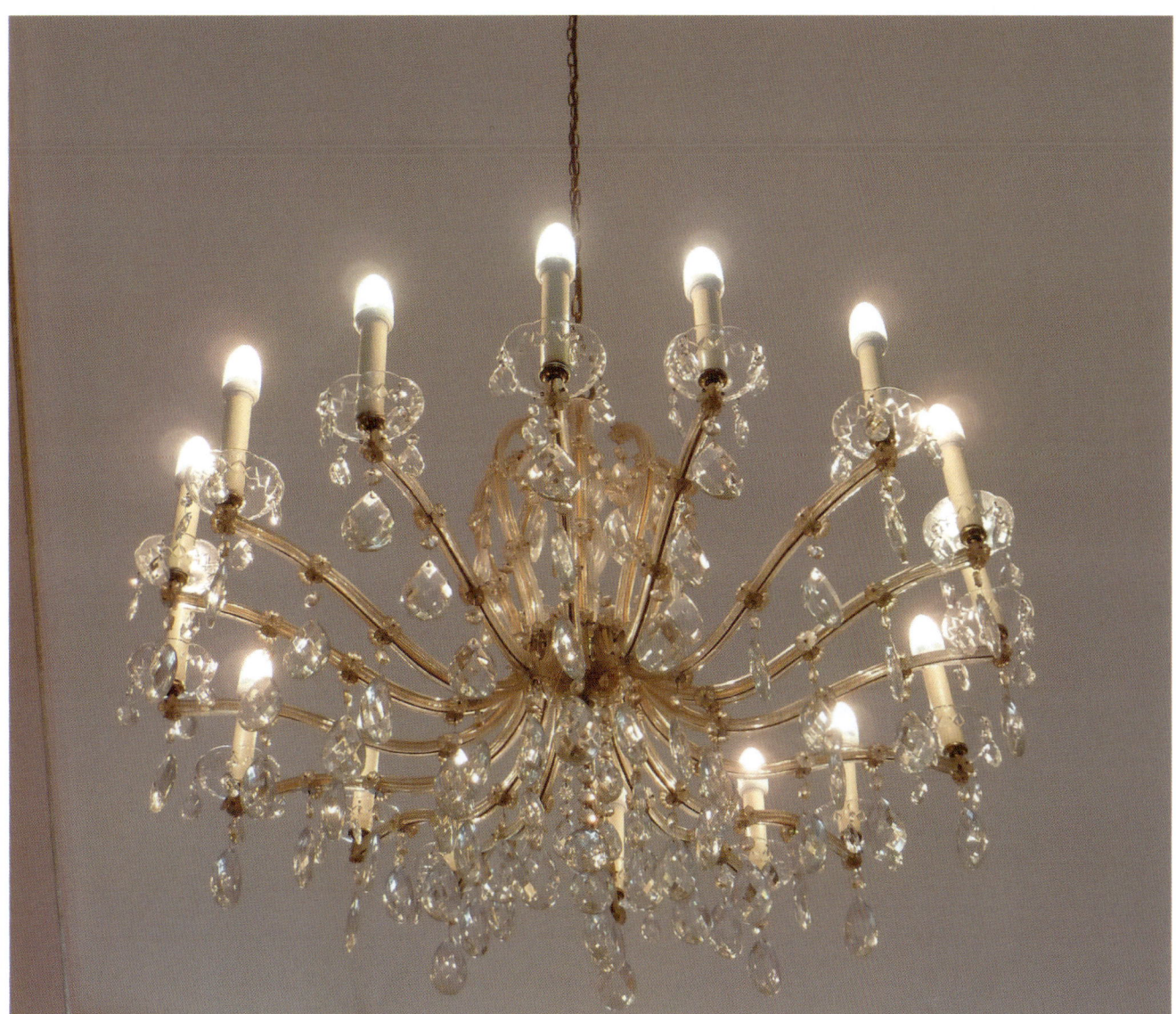

1. That is a beautiful crystal _____.

2. Where would you find it?

3. Who has them?

4. When do you use one?

5. Explain how to clean one.

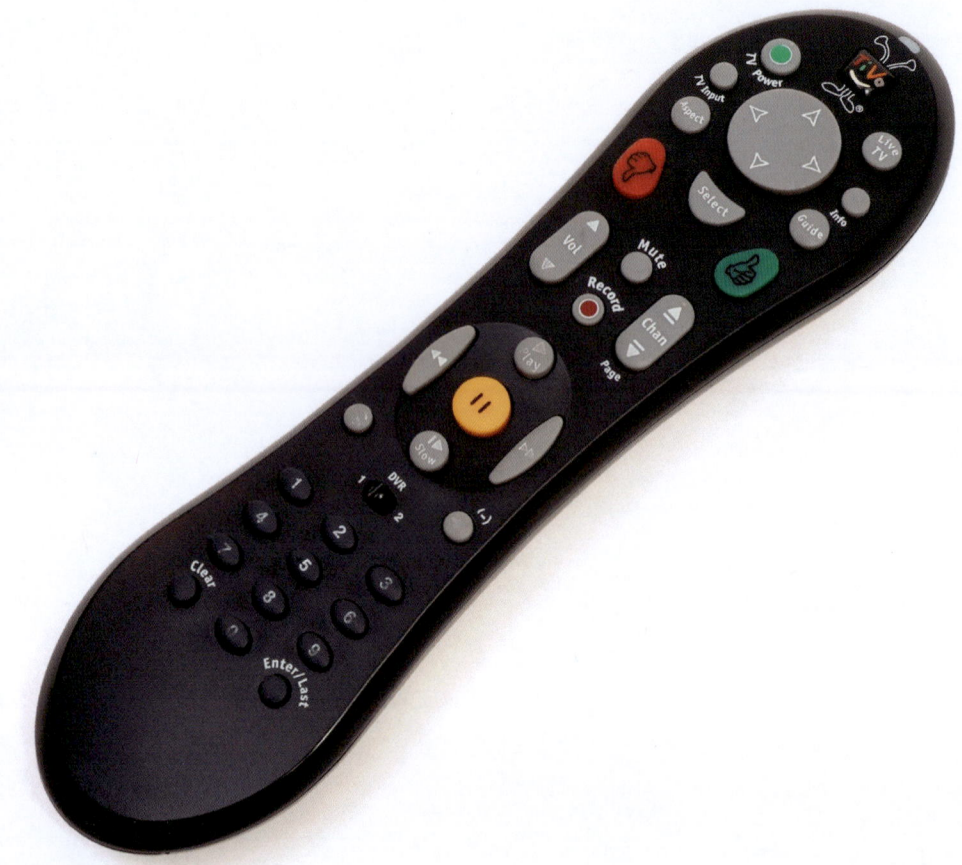

1.   Look under the couch cushion. I can't find the _____.

2.   Where do you find one?

3.   Who uses it?

4.   What is it for?

5.   Pretend like you are using one.

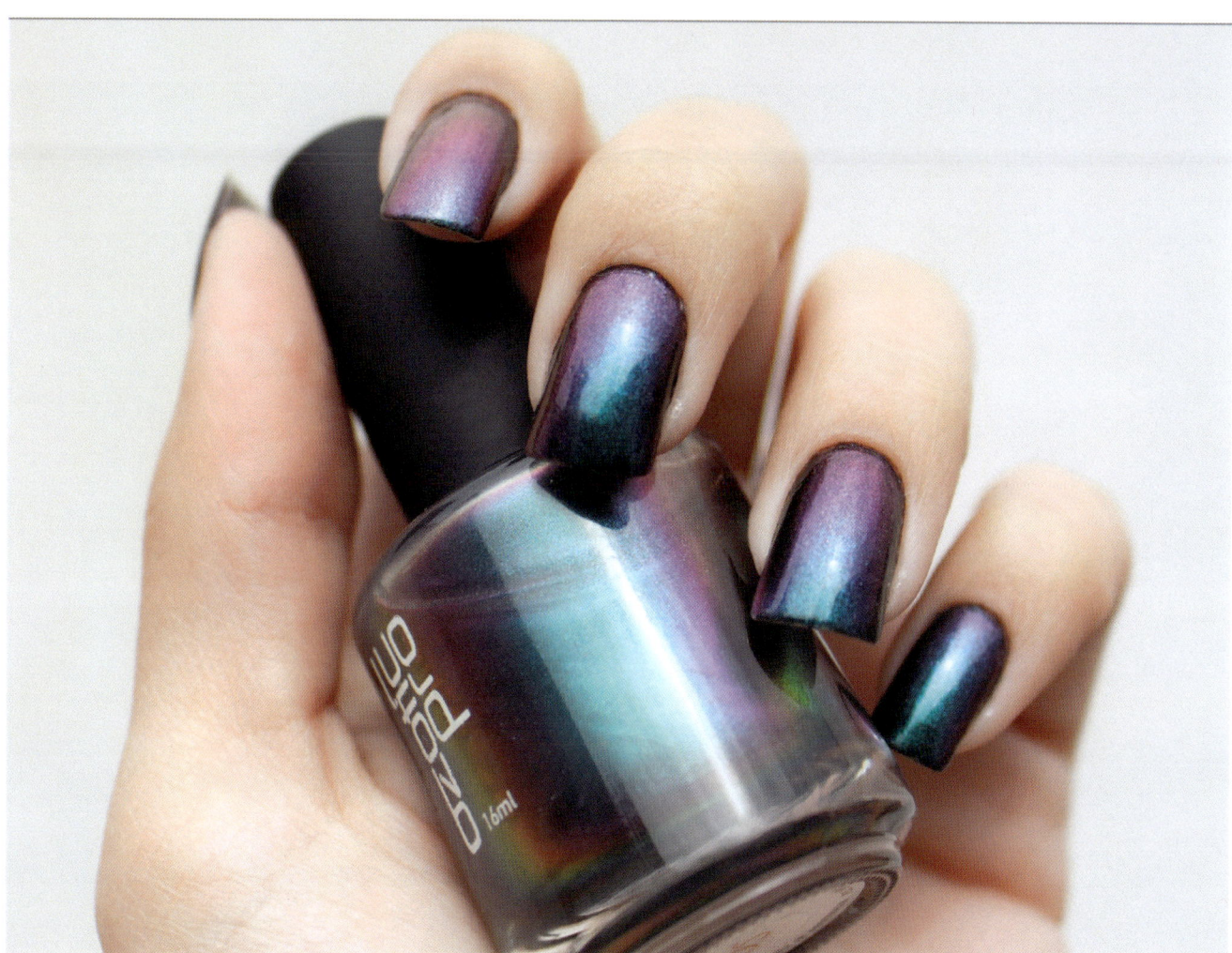

1.   That is a pretty bottle of nail _____.

2.   Where do you purchase it?

3.   Who uses it?

4.   What is it for?

5.   Pretend like you are painting your nails.

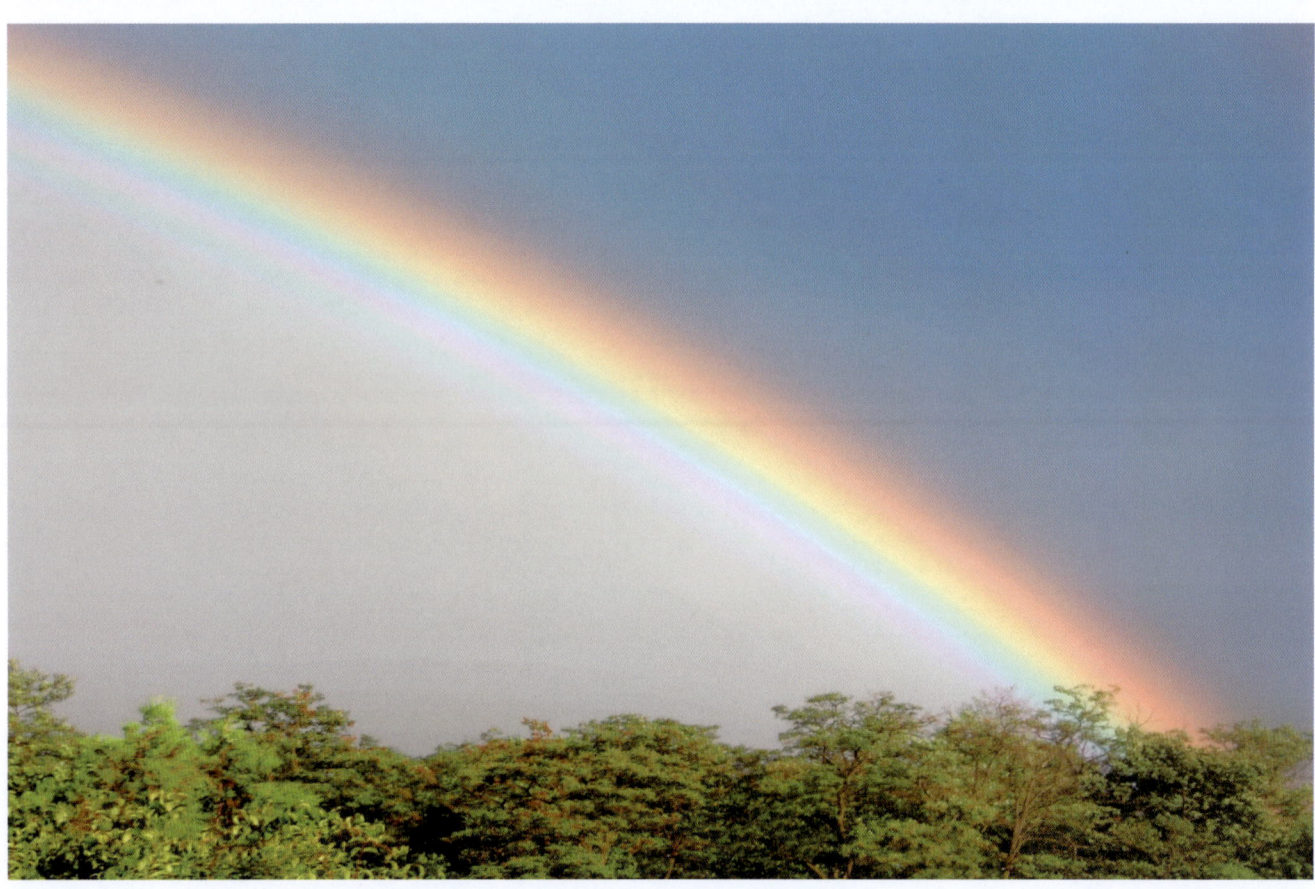

xvii

1. Somewhere over the _____.

2. What are the colors in a rainbow?

3. When do you see them?

4. Why do they appear?

5. Sing "Somewhere Over the Rainbow."

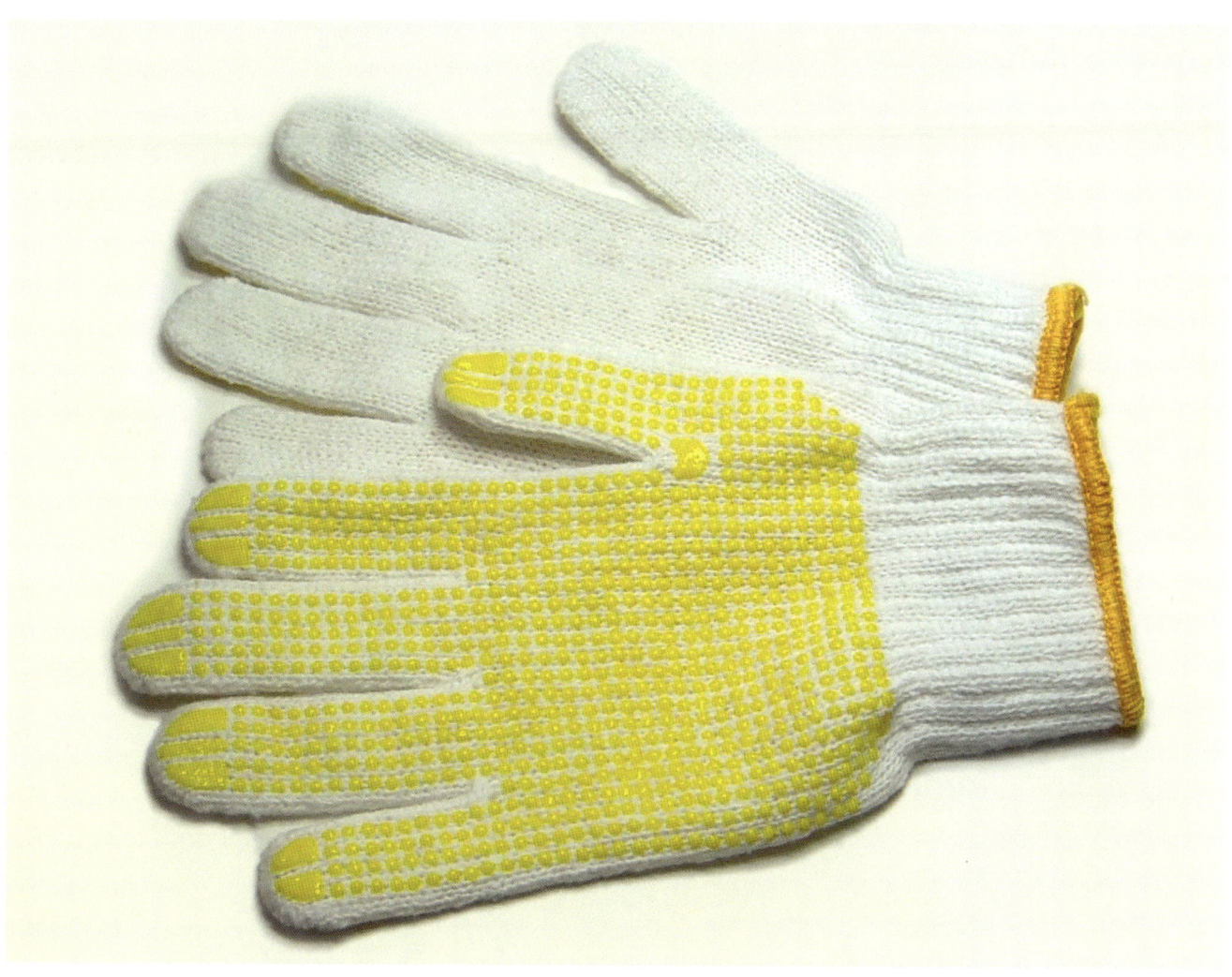

xviii

1. My hands are cold I wish I had a pair of _____.

2. What do you put them on?

3. When do you wear them?

4. Why would you wear them.

5. Pretend you are putting on a pair.

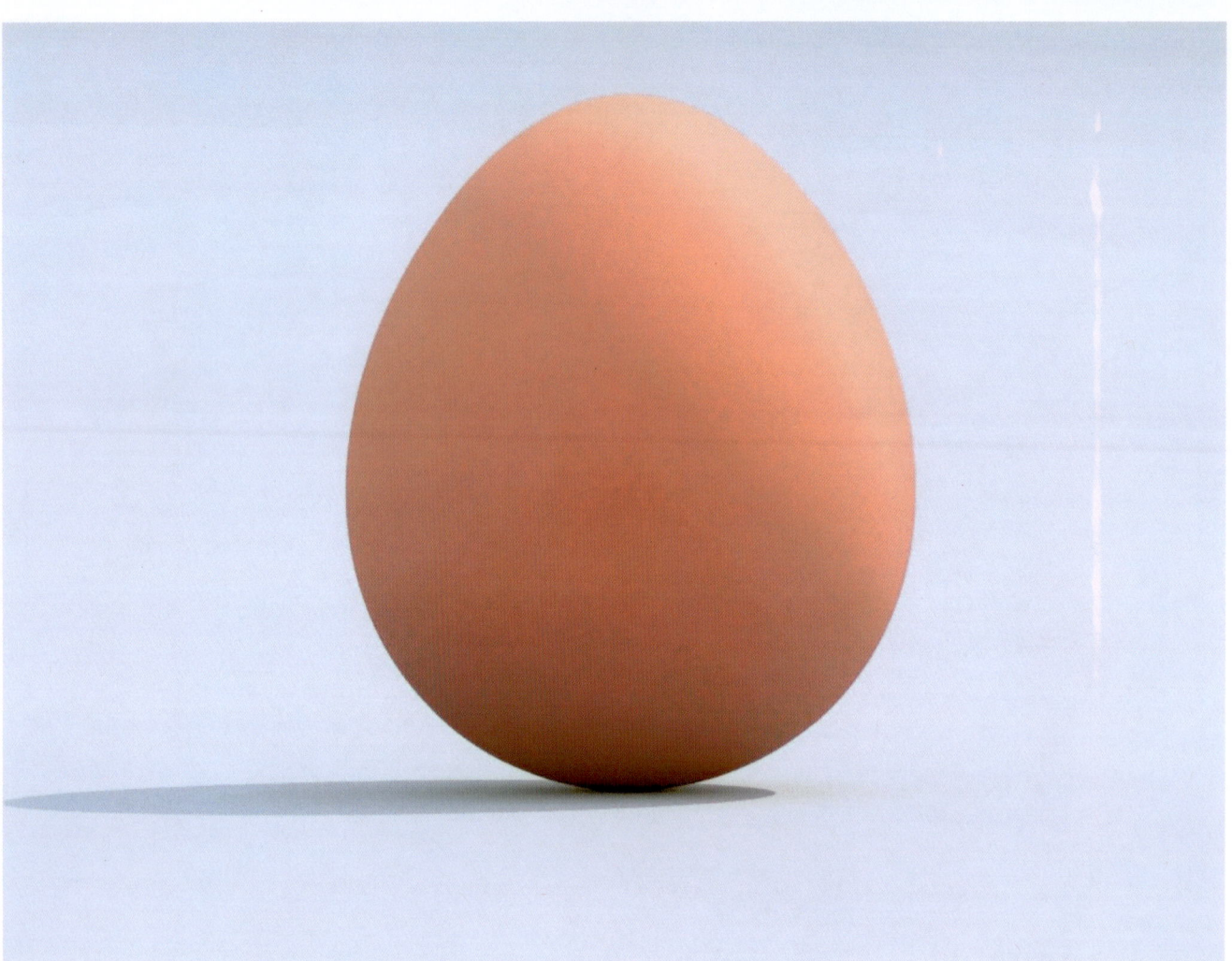

xix

1. I'd like a hard boiled _____.

2. What colors can they be?

3. What different ways can you cook them?

4. What time of day do you eat them?

5. Pretend you are cracking one.

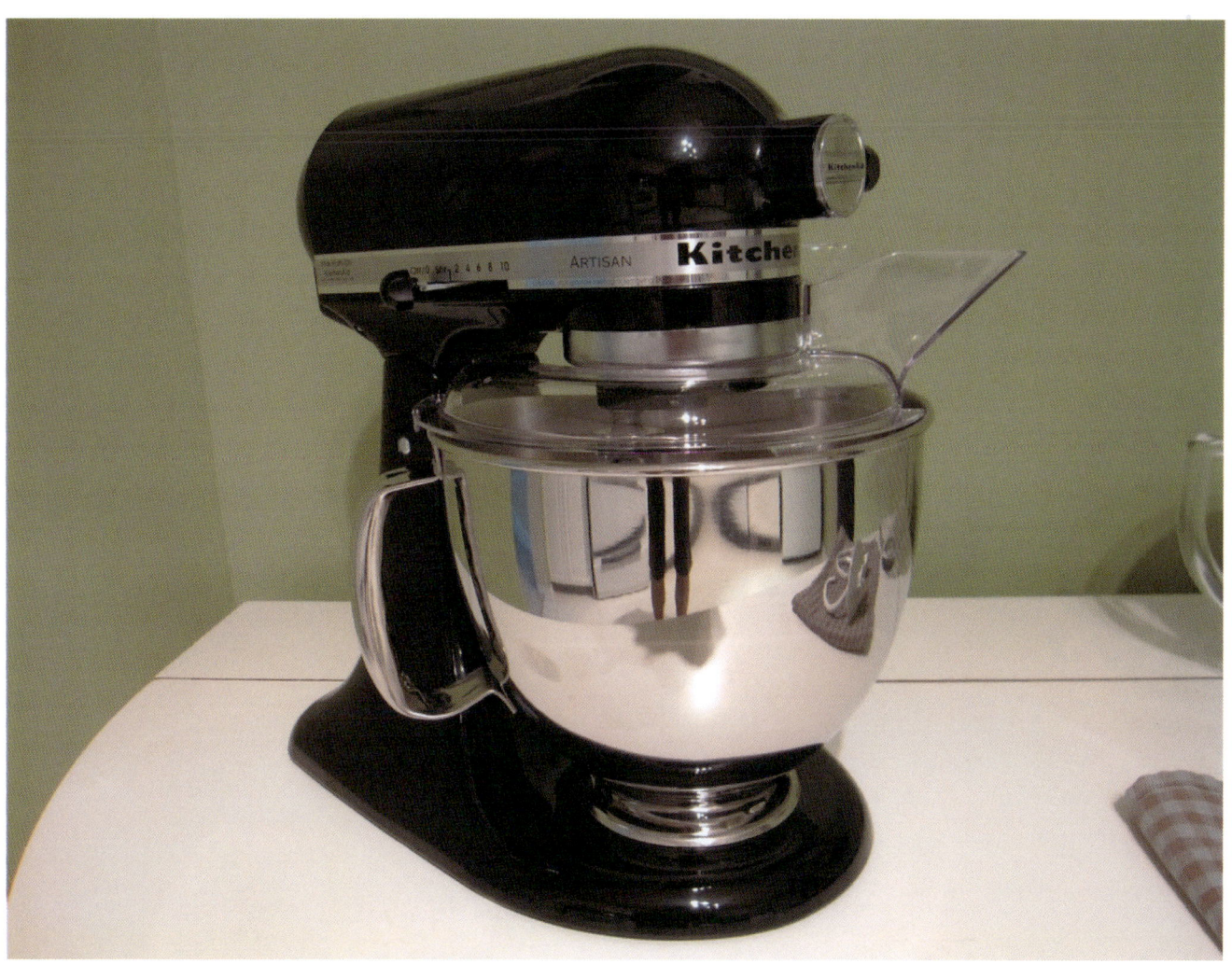

xx

1.   I'm making a cake and will use my new electric _____.

2.   Where do you keep it?

3.   What is it used for?

4.   How much do you think it costs?

5.   Make a sound imitating it.

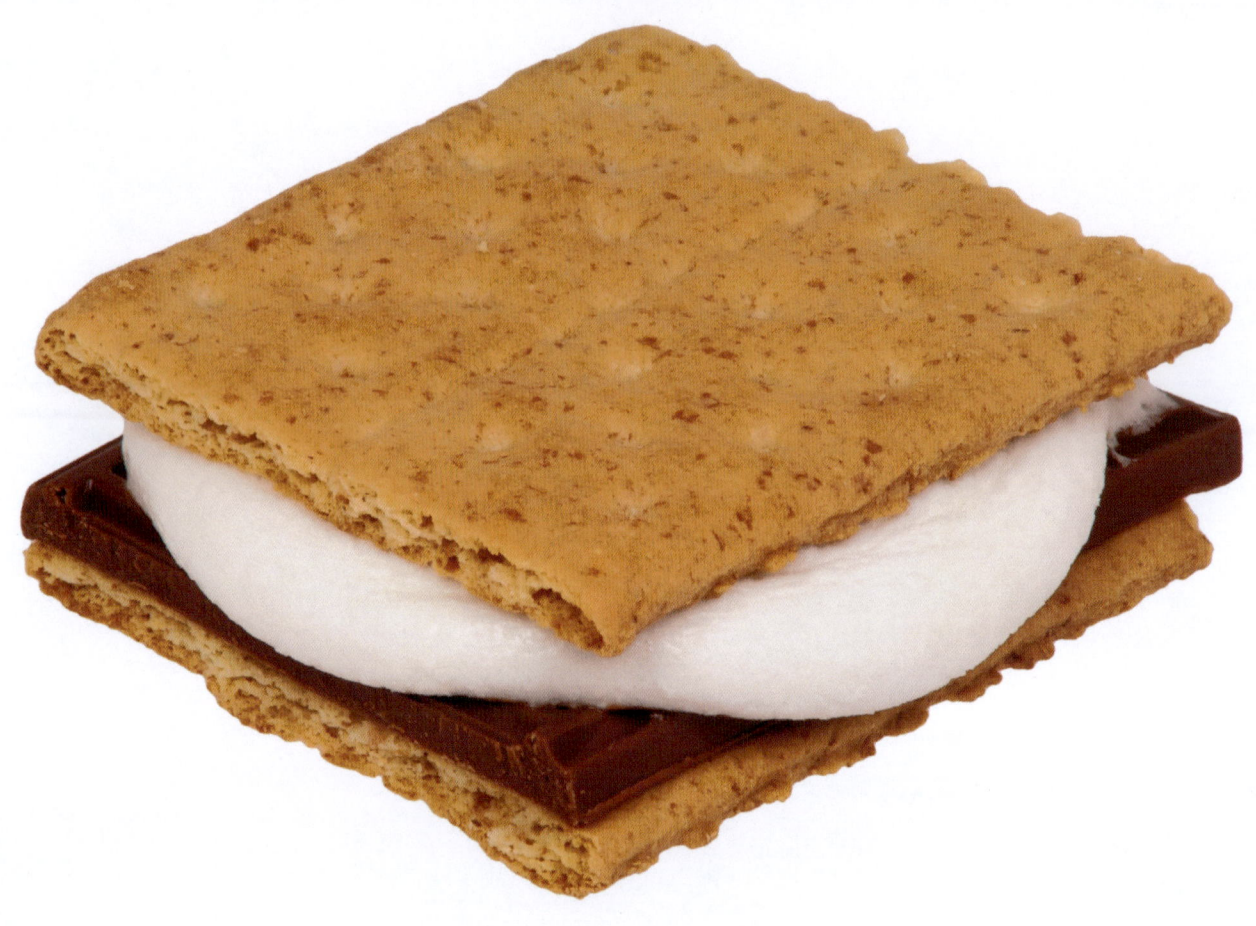

1.   My favorite summer treat is a _____.

2.   What are the ingredients?

3.   How do you make one?

4.   Where would you make one?

5.   Pretend to toast a marshmallow.

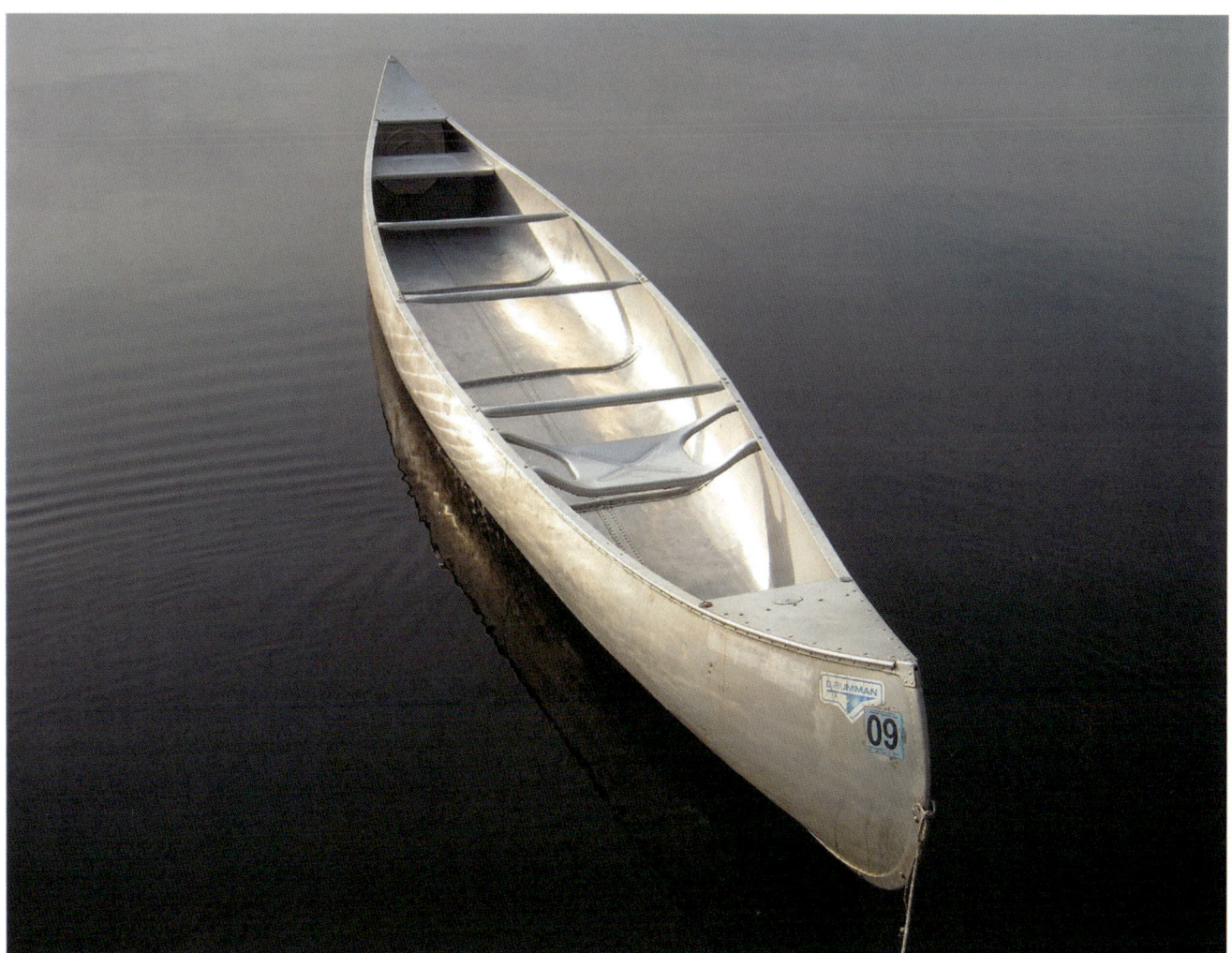

1.   Would you like to go for a ride in the _____.

2.   Where would you use it?

3.   How do you propel it?

4.   What would you wear when you were in one?

5.   Pretend you are in one.

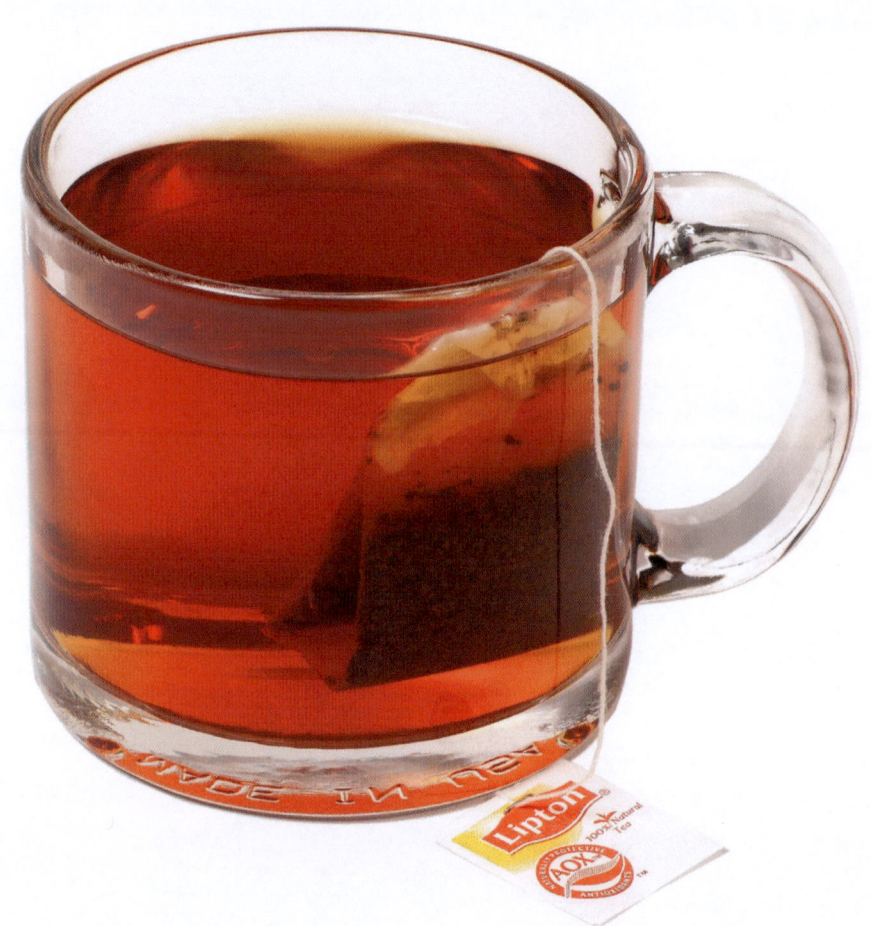

1.   I like to drink English Breakfast _____.

2.   When do people drink it?

3.   Who drinks it?

4.   Where do you find it?

5.   Pretend you are drinking some.

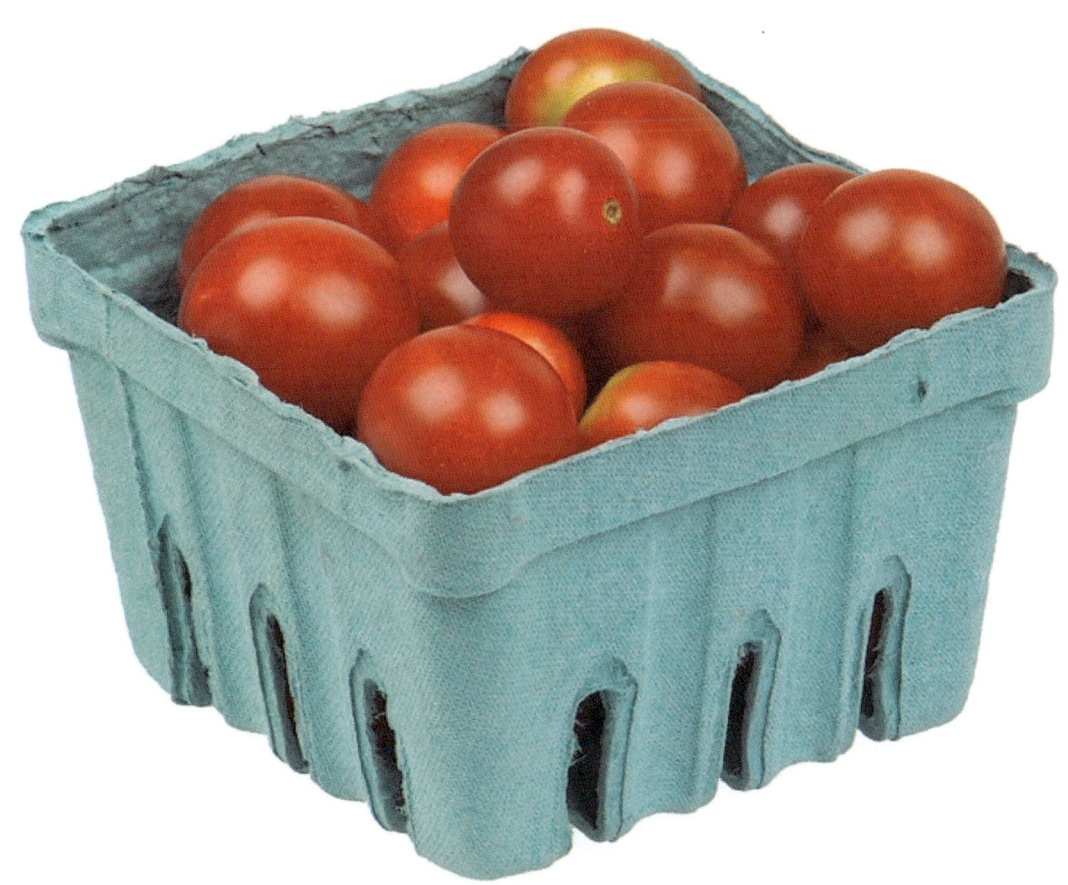

1.   Salad is delicious with cherry _____.

2.   Where do you keep them?

3.   When do they grow?

4.   How do you feel about them?

5.   Pretend you are eating one.

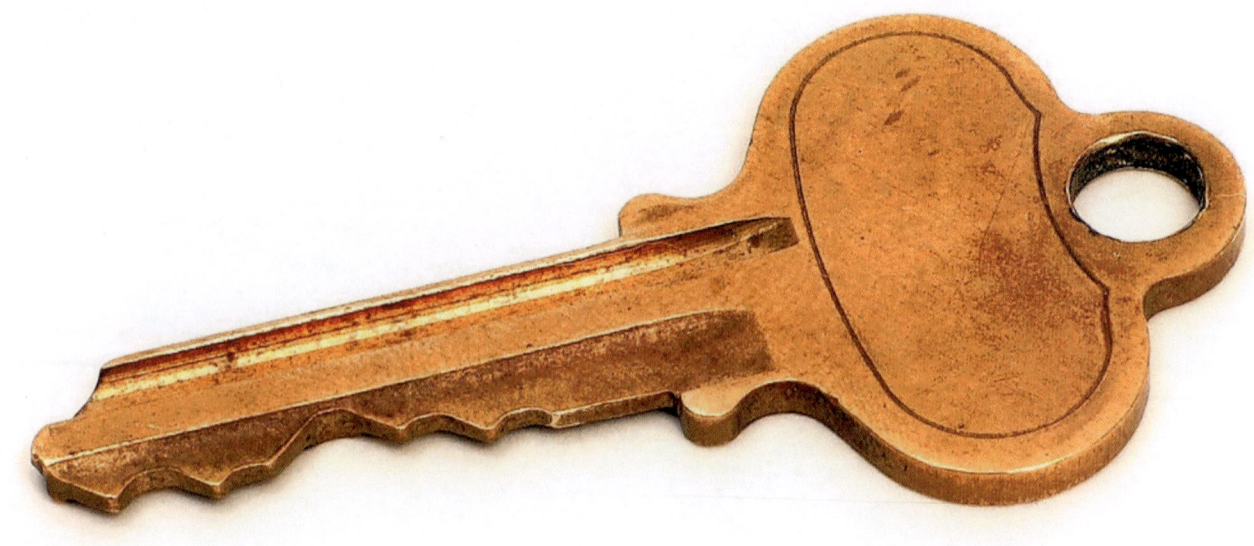

xxv

1. I'm going to be late! I can't find my _____.

2. Where do you keep them?

3. What is it for?

4. What things do you need one for?

5. Pretend you are using one.

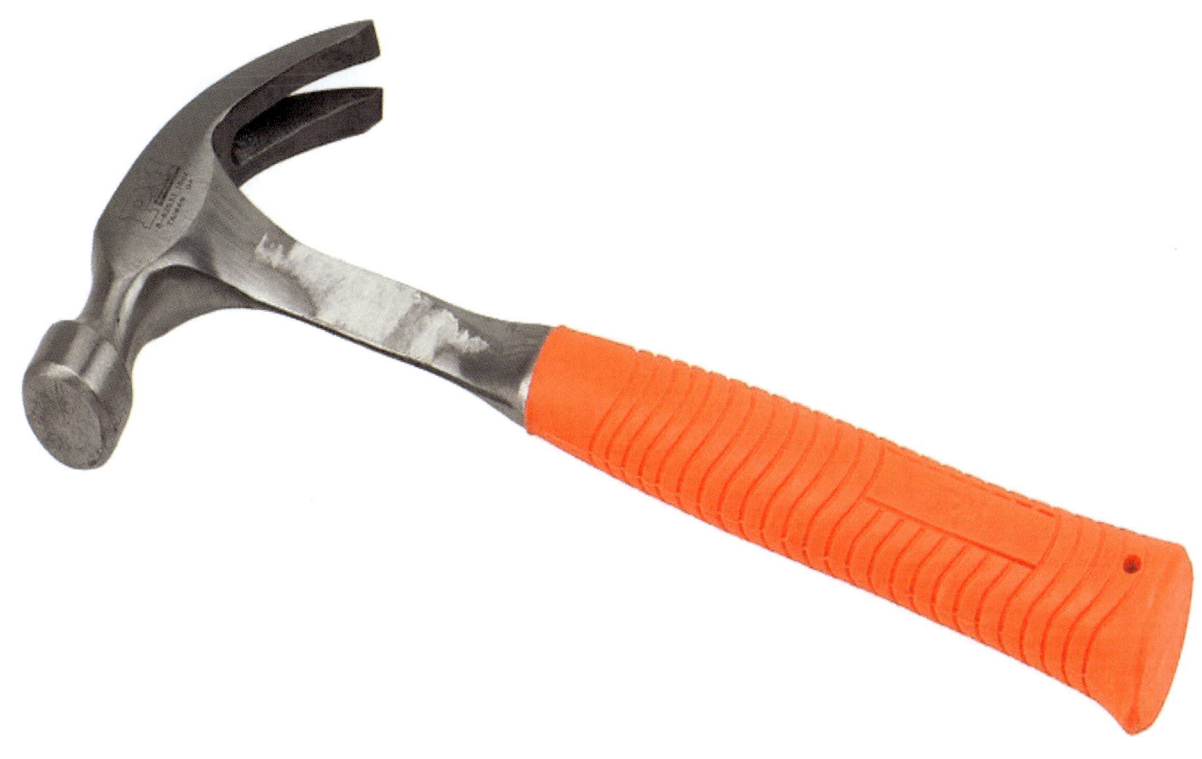

1.   I'm going to hit this nail with my _____.

2.   Where do you keep it?

3.   Who uses it?

4.   What do you do with it?

5.   Pretend you are using one.

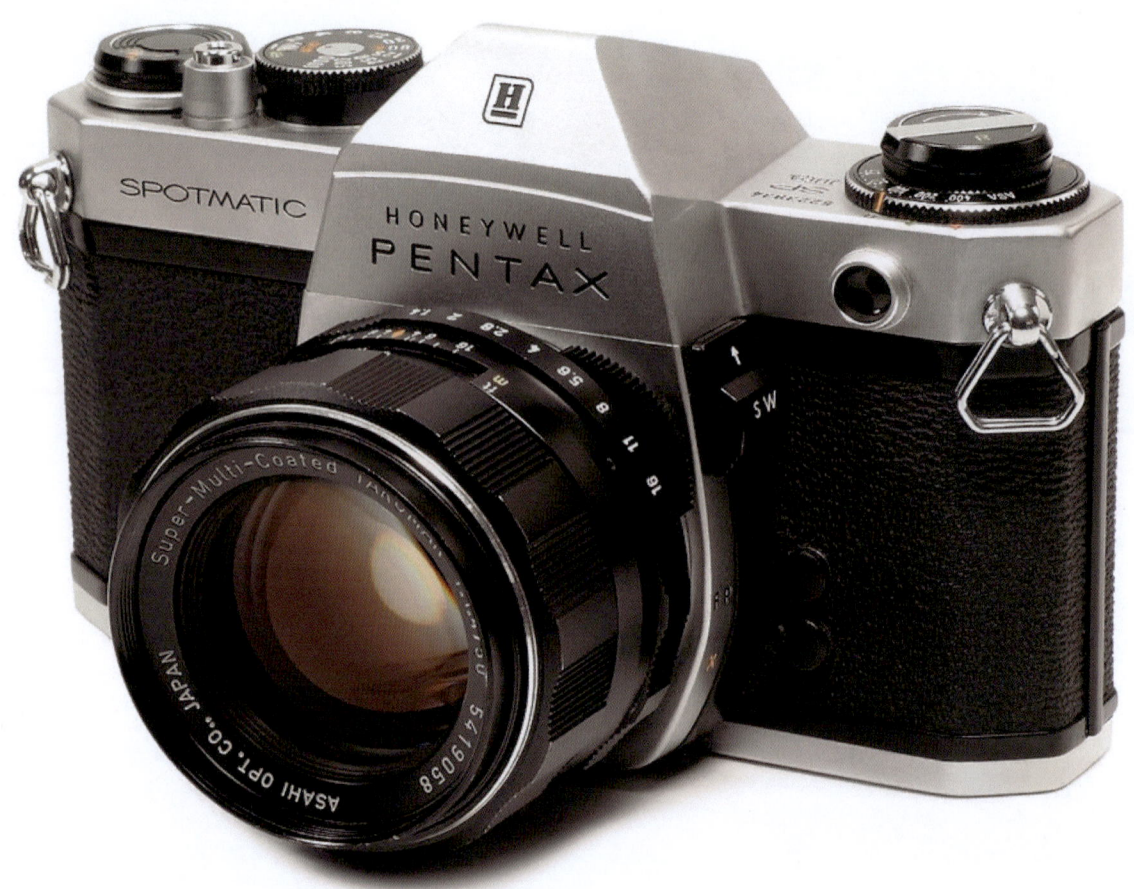

1. I'm going to take a picture with my _____.

2. What events would you use one?

3. What does it do?

4. Who uses them professionally?

5. Pretend you are taking a picture.

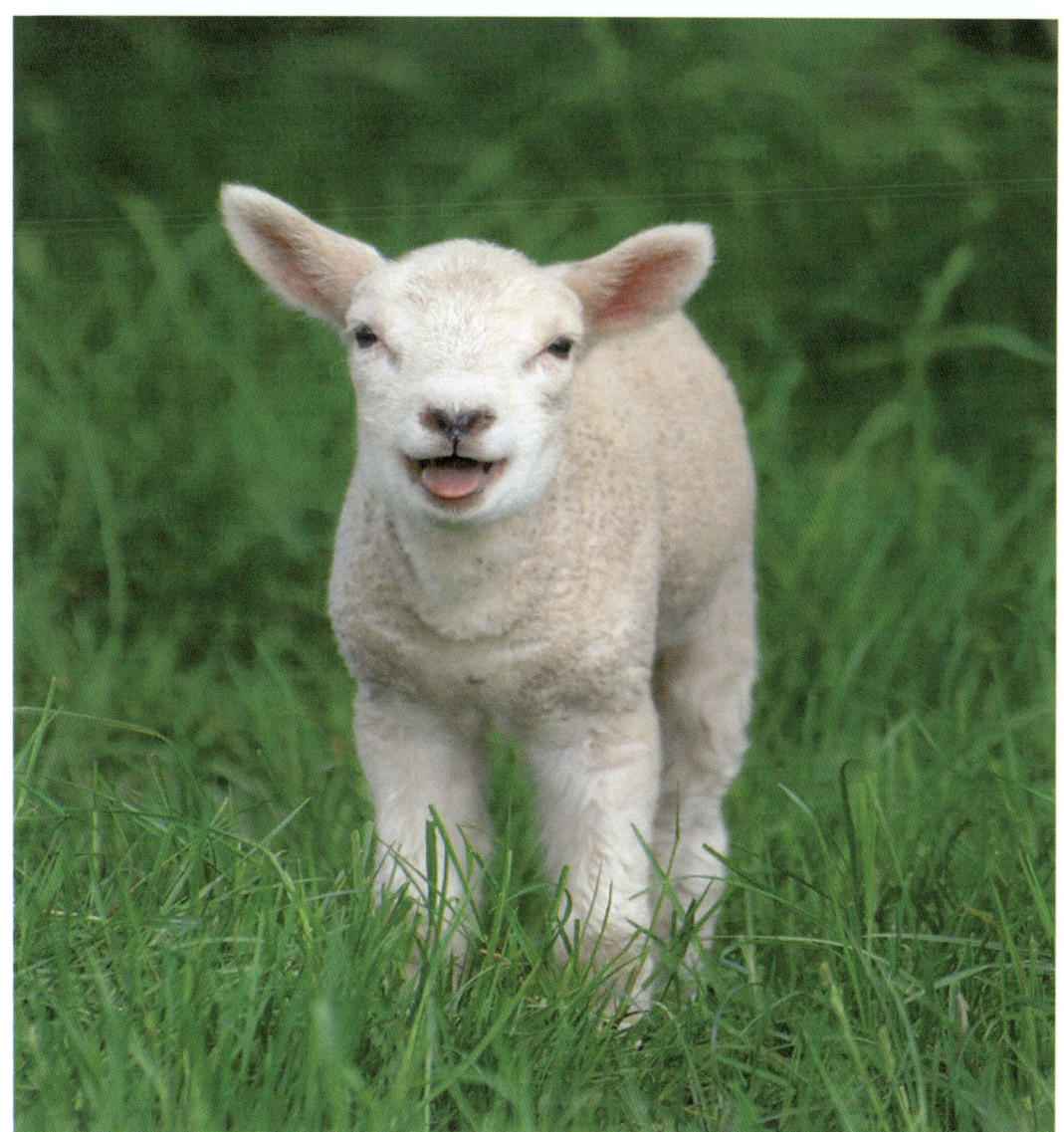

1. A baby sheep is called a _____.

2. What is their fur called?

3. What is it used for?

4. Where would you find a lamb?

5. Sing "Mary had a little lamb"

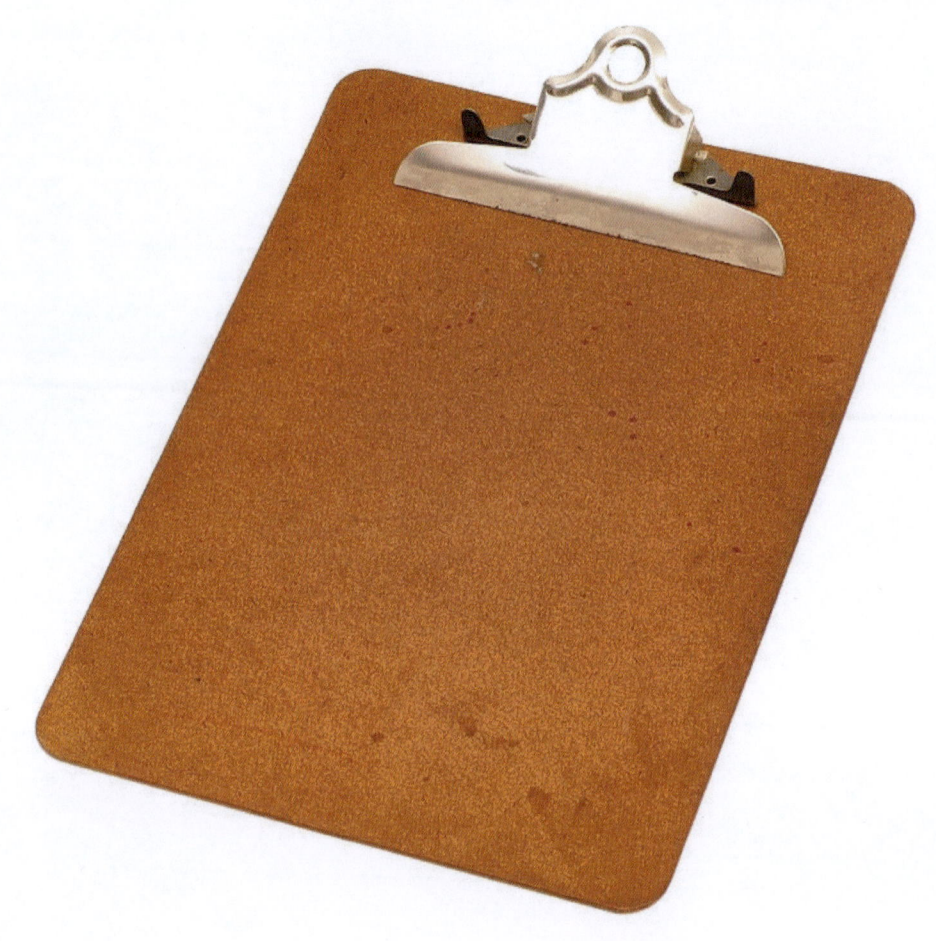

1. Take notes using this _____.

2. Who uses one?

3. What is it used for?

4. What do you put on it?

5. Pretend you are writing with one.

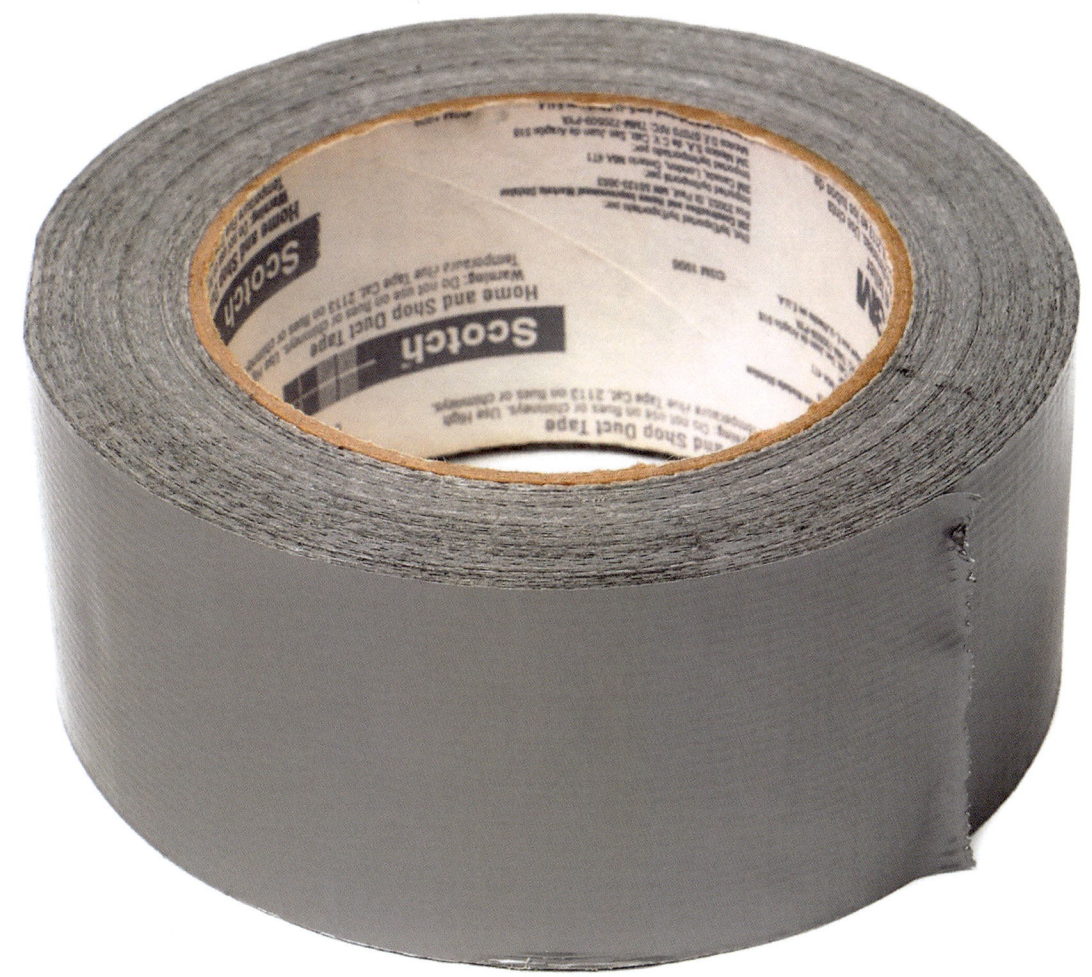

1.   The couch was worn and covered in _____.

2.   What do you use it for?

3.   Who uses it?

4.   Where would you put it?

5.   Make the sound it makes when you unroll it.

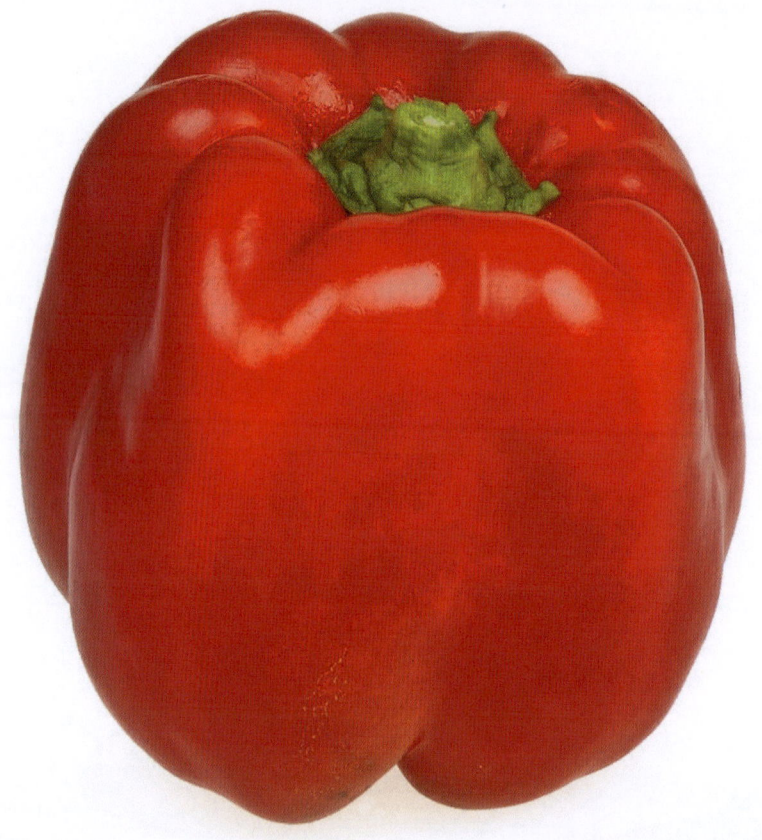

xxx

1. I'll have a chicken fajita with sauteed onions and red _____ .

2. What other colors do they come in?

3. Where could you buy them?

4. What dishes do you serve them in?

5. Pretend you slicing one with a knife.

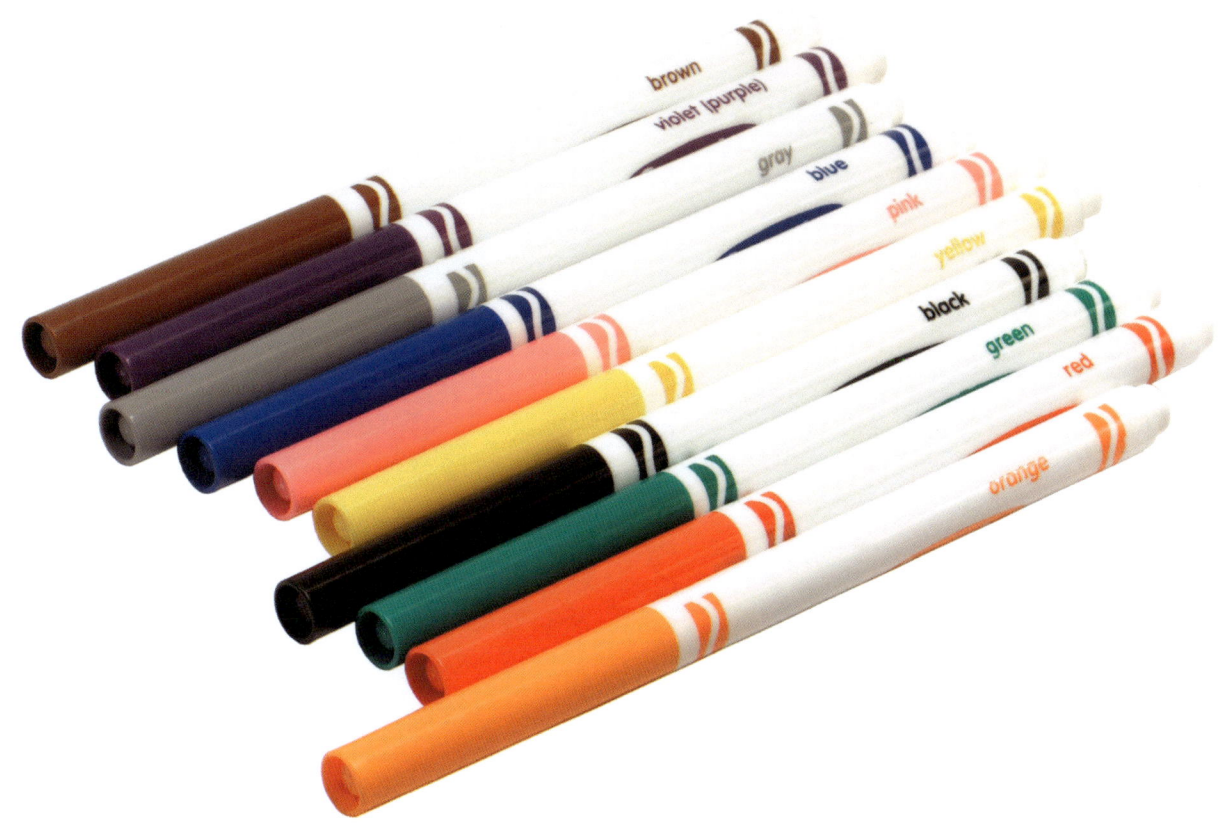

xxxi

1. I'm going to draw a picture with these colored _____.

2. What colors do they come in?

3. Who uses them?

4. Where would you find them?

5. What would you draw with them?

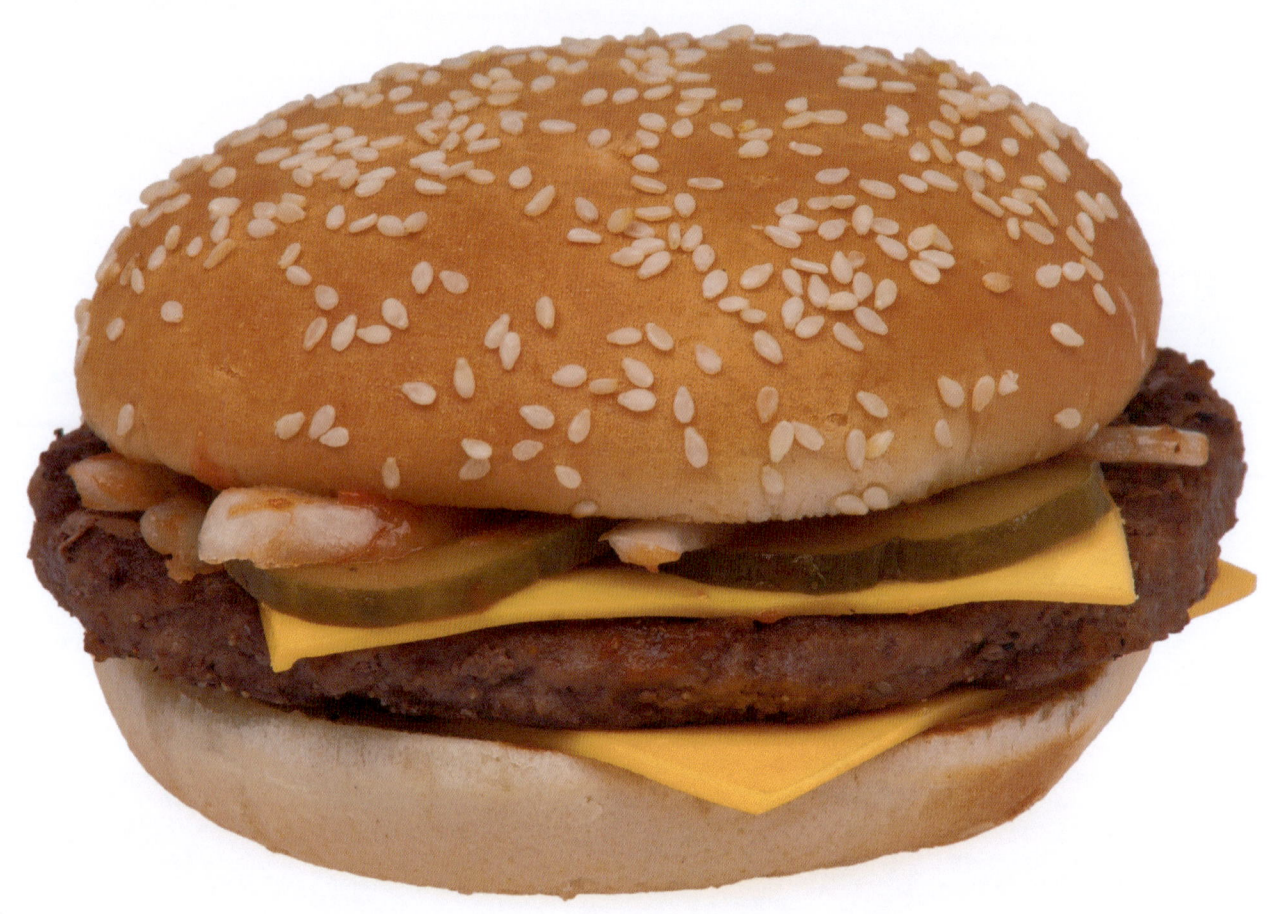

1. I like pickles and onions on my cheese _____.

2. Where could you buy one?

3. When would you eat one?

4. Why shouldn't you eat one?

5. What could you put on one?

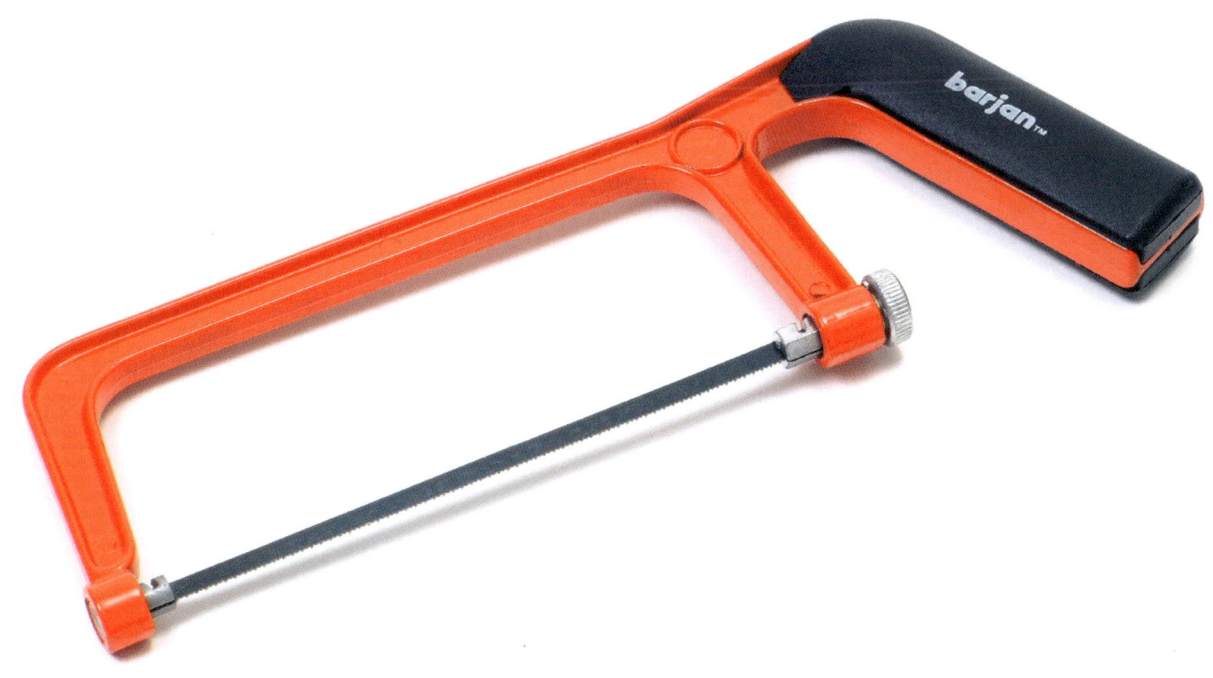

1.   I asked to borrow my neighbor's hack _____.

2.   Where would you keep it?

3.   What would you use it for?

4.   Who would use it?

5.   Pretend you are using one.

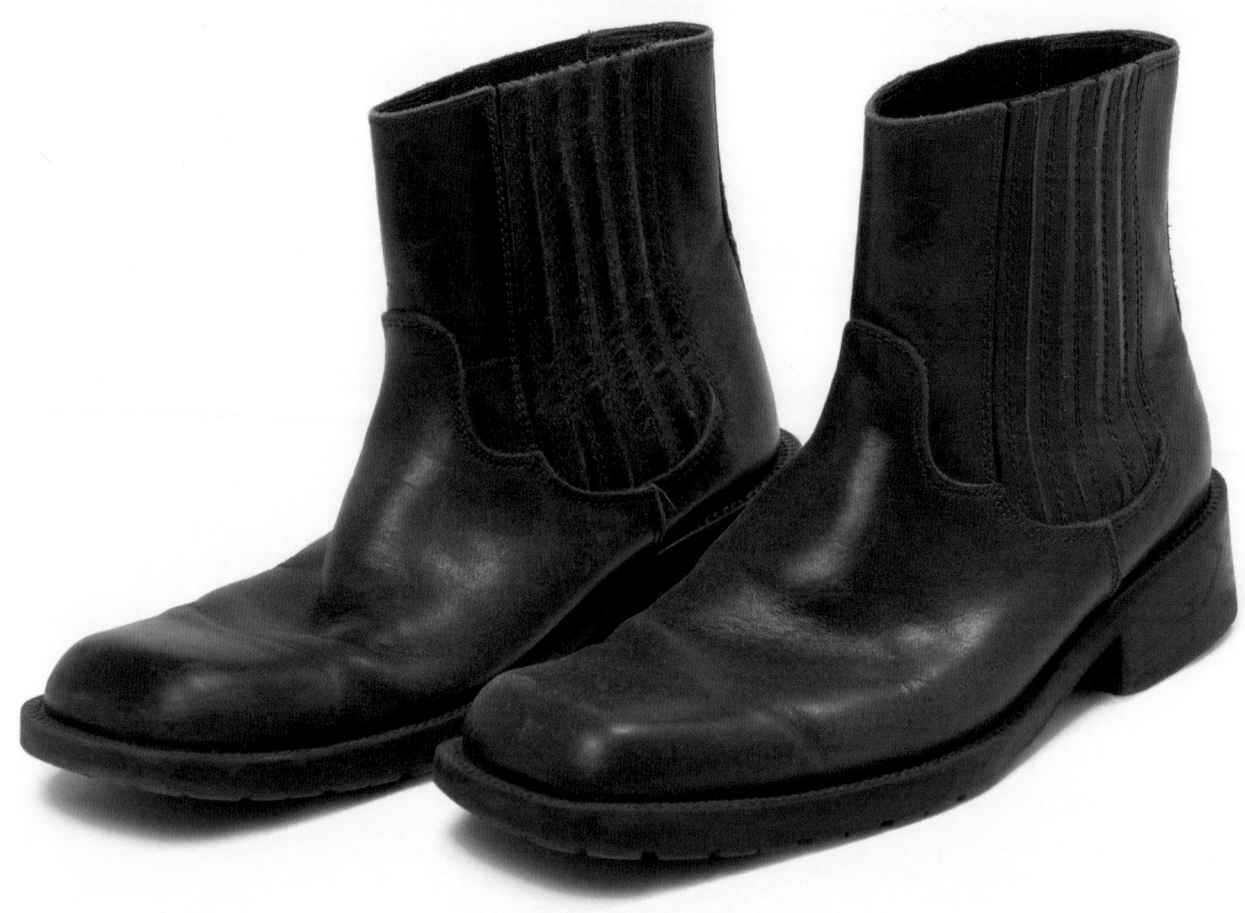

xxxiv

1. I need a pair of leather _____.

2. Who would wear these?

3. When would they wear these?

4. What do you put them on?

5. Sing a verse from "These boots are made for walking."

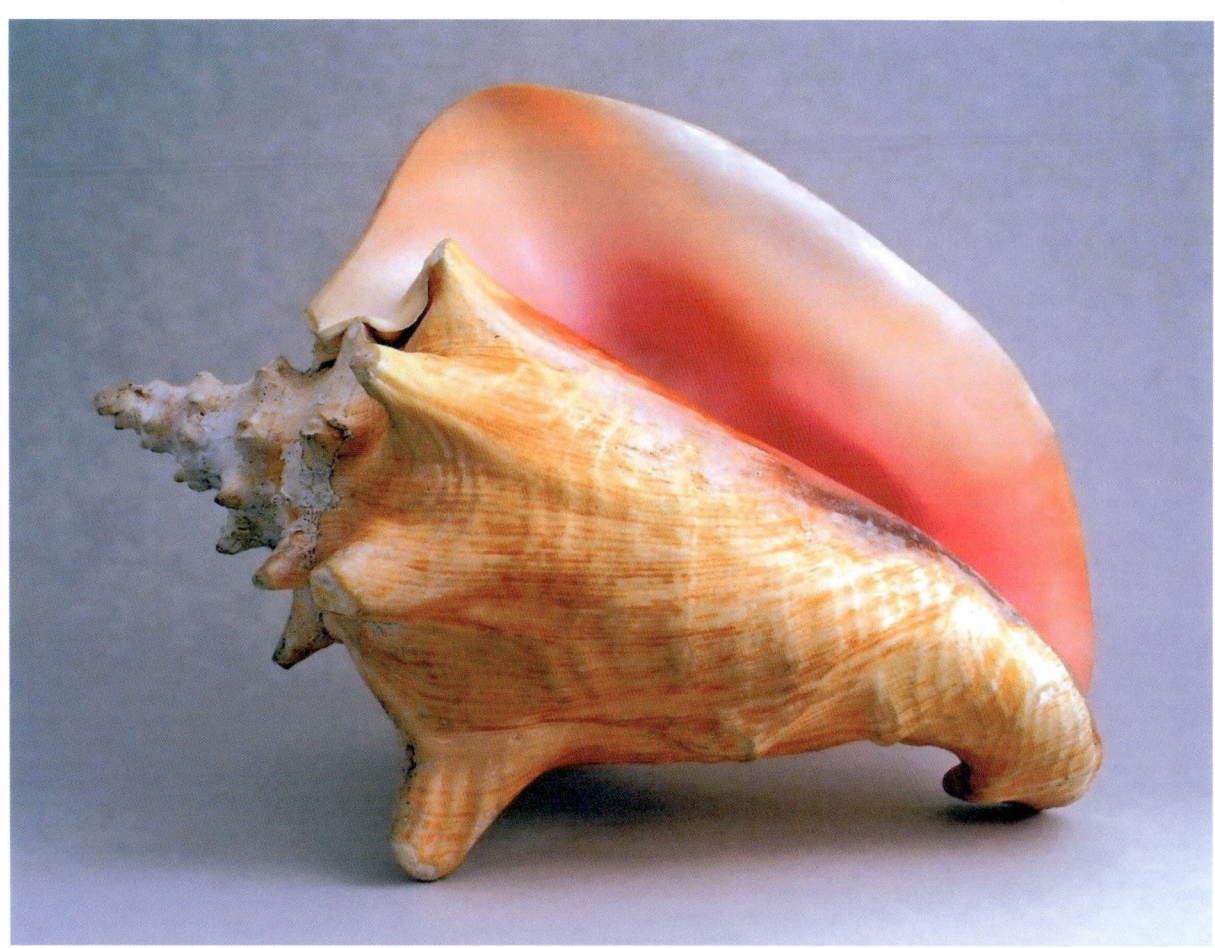

xxxv

1. Wow, what a beautiful sea _____.

2. Where do you find it?

3. What can you do with it?

4. What lives inside of it?

5. Pretend you are blowing into one.

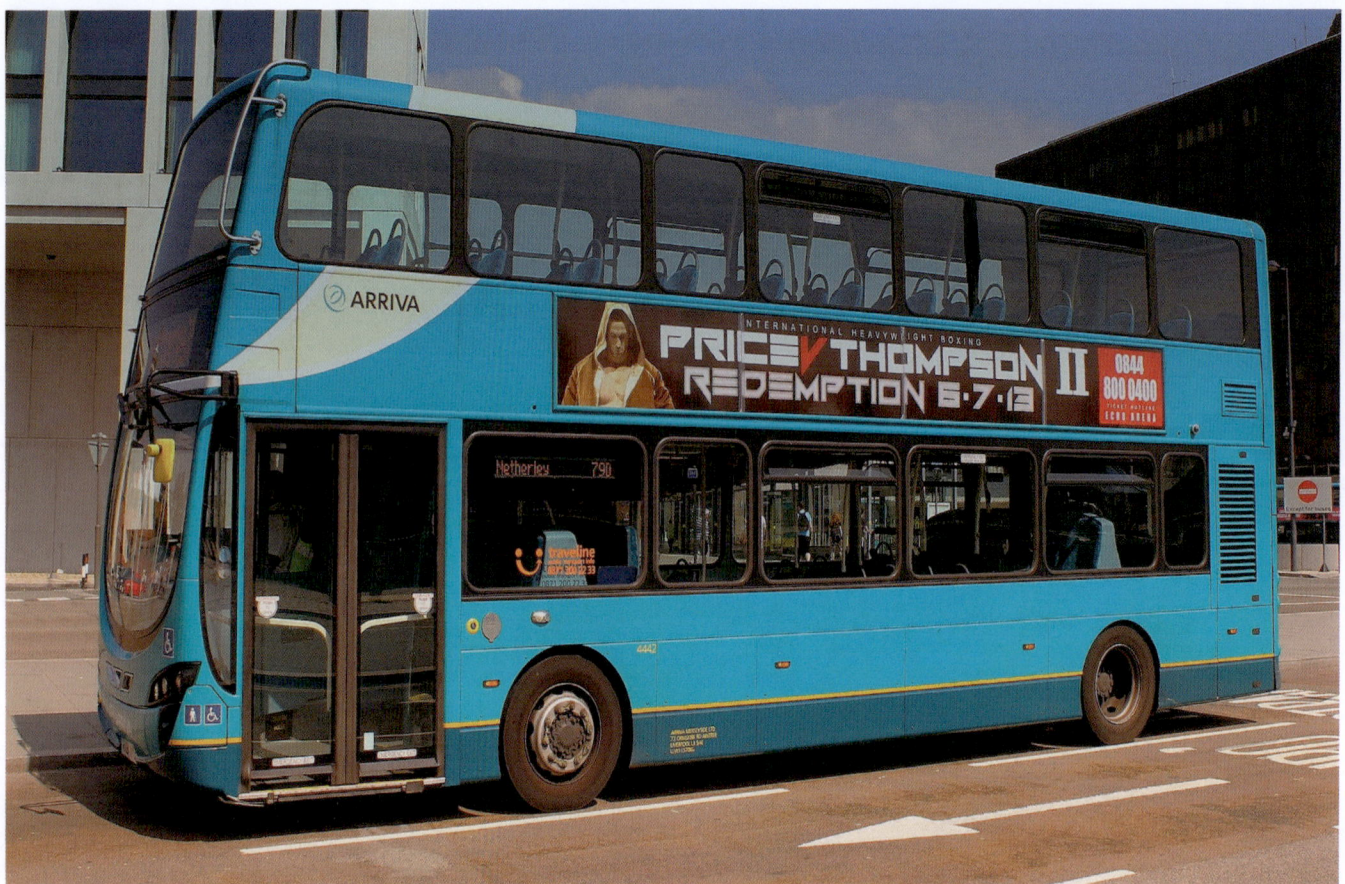

xxxvi

1. I'm waiting for the _____.

2. What kind of bus is this?

3. Where would you see one?

4. Why would you ride one?

5. Sing "The wheels on the bus go round and round."

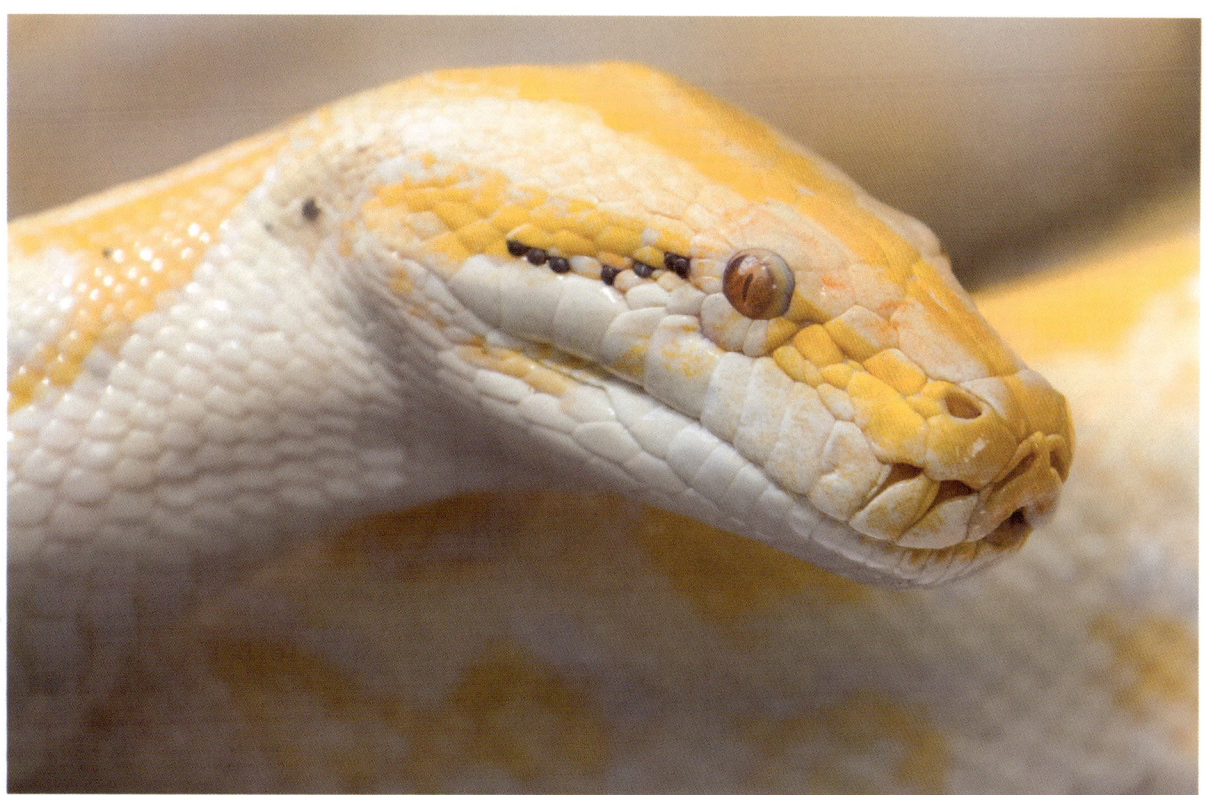

xxxvii

1. I am terrified of _____.

2. Where do they live?

3. What do they eat?

4. Why are they dangerous?

5. Make a sound like one.

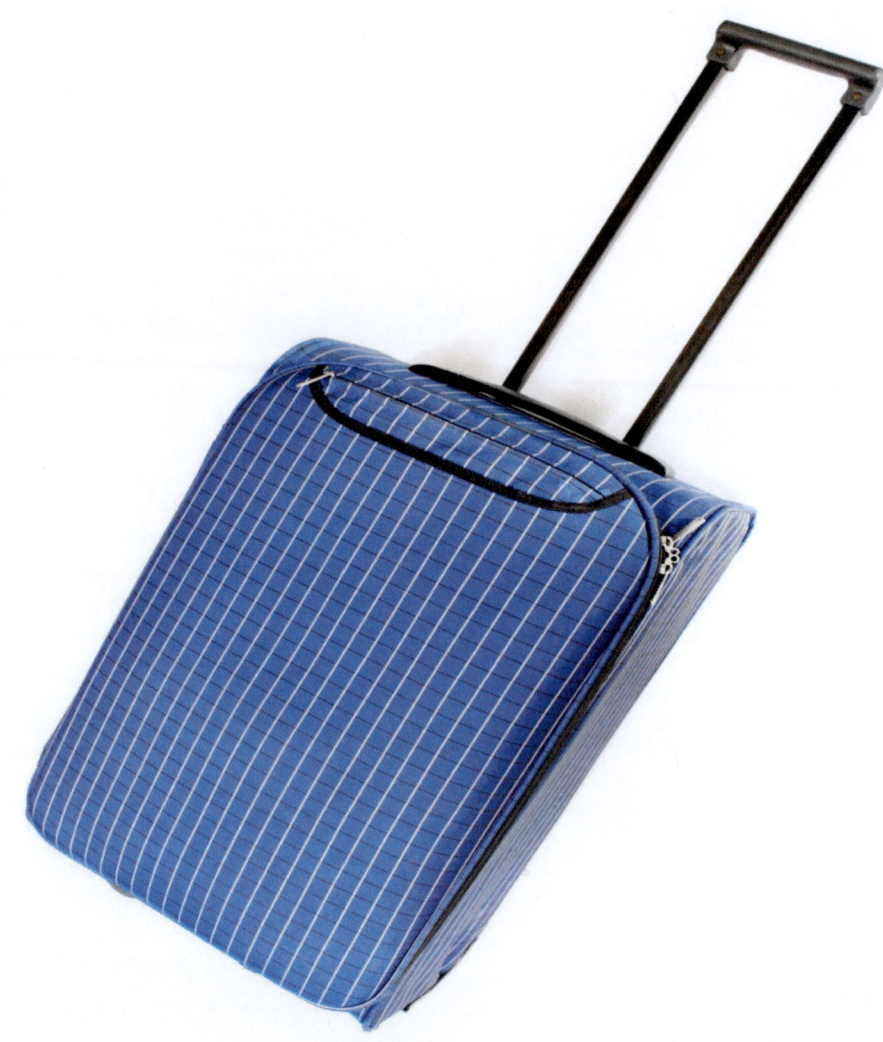

1.   I'm going on a trip. I need to pack my _____.

2.   What do you put in it?

3.   Where do you take it?

4.   When do you need one?

5.   Pretend you are packing.

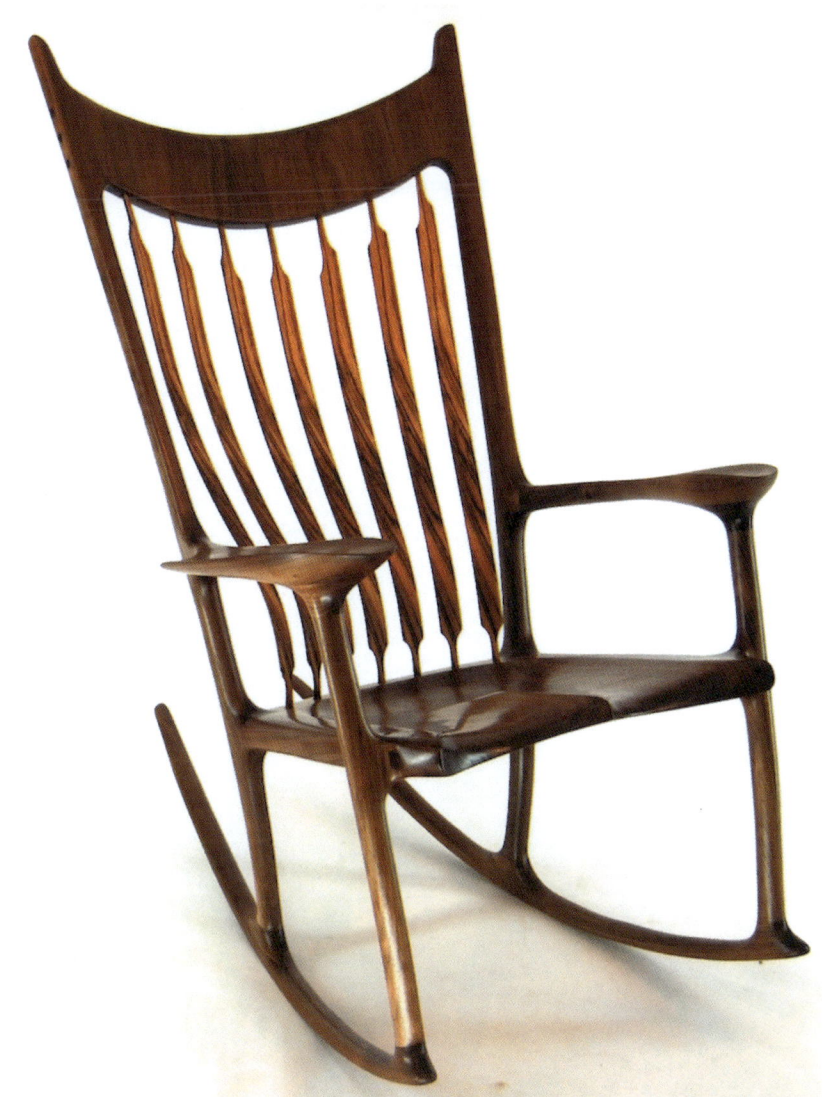

1. I'm going to sit down in this rocking _____.

2. Who uses them?

3. What do you do with one?

4. Where would you find one?

5. Pretend you are sitting in one.

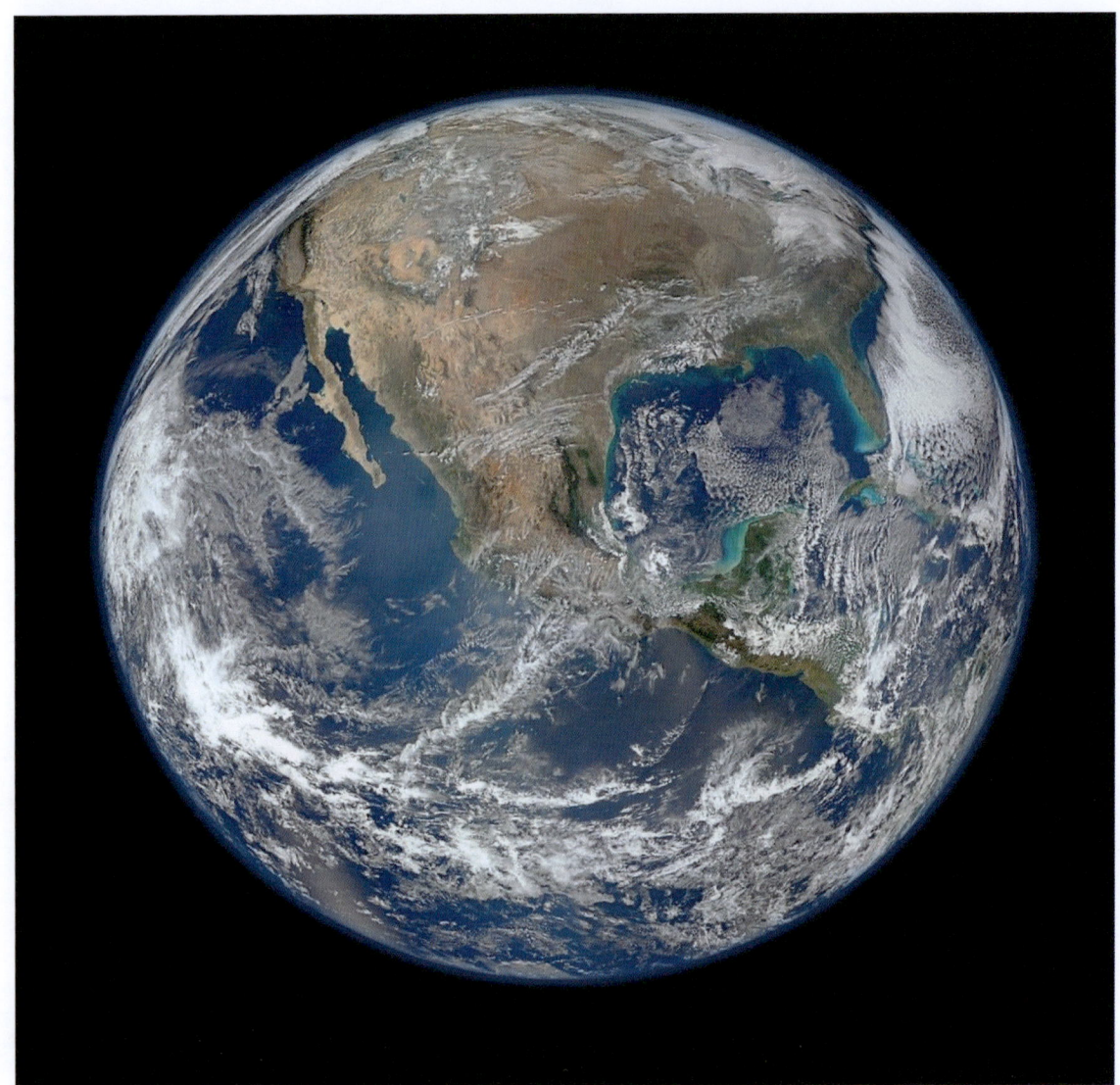

xl

1.	We live on the planet _____.

2.	What continent is showing?

3.	Where is the photo taken from?

4.	What shape is Earth?

5.	Name three other planets.

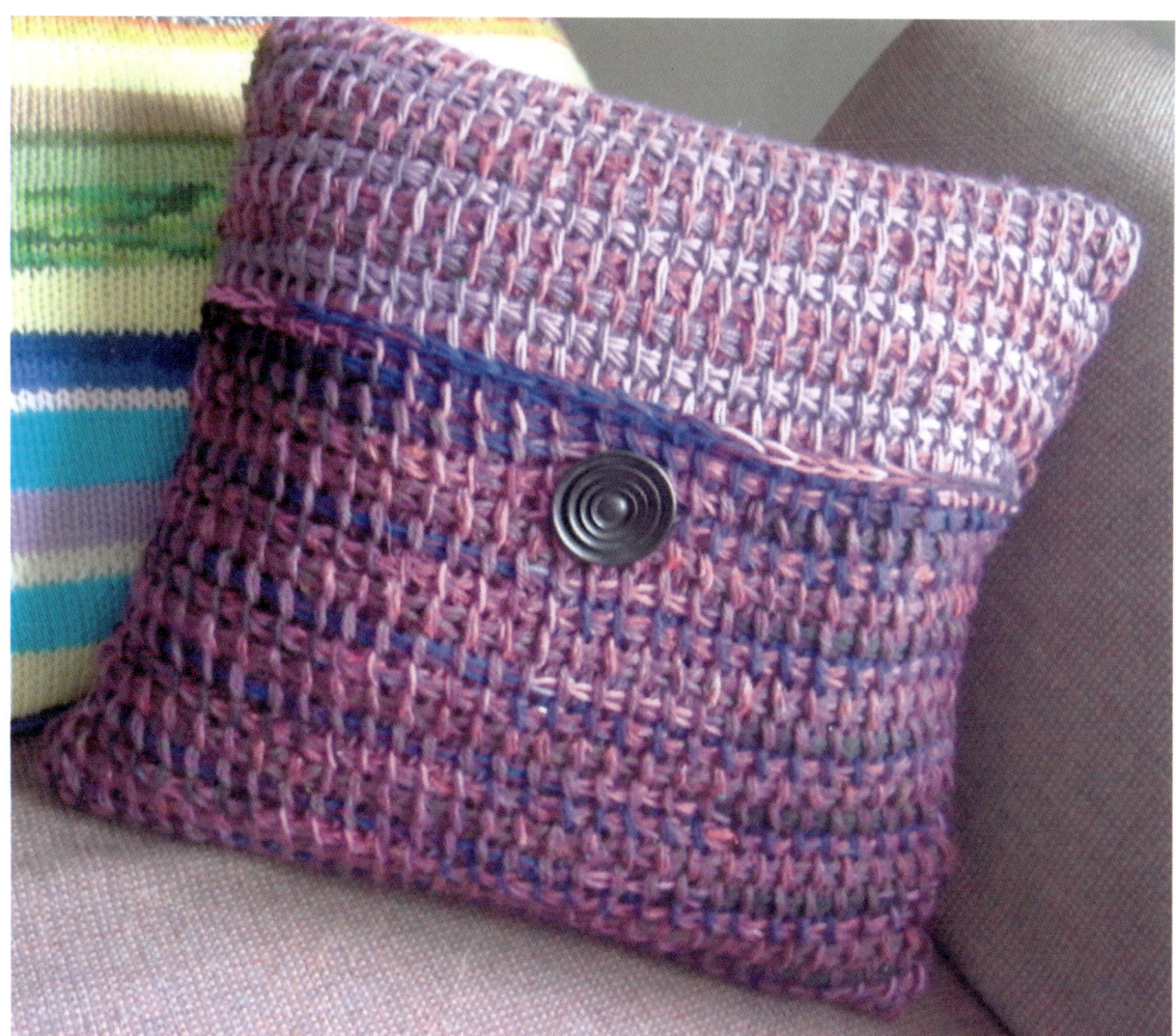

1. That is a pretty purple _____.

2. Where do you put one?

3. What do you do with it?

4. How was this one made?

5. What kind of pillow is this?

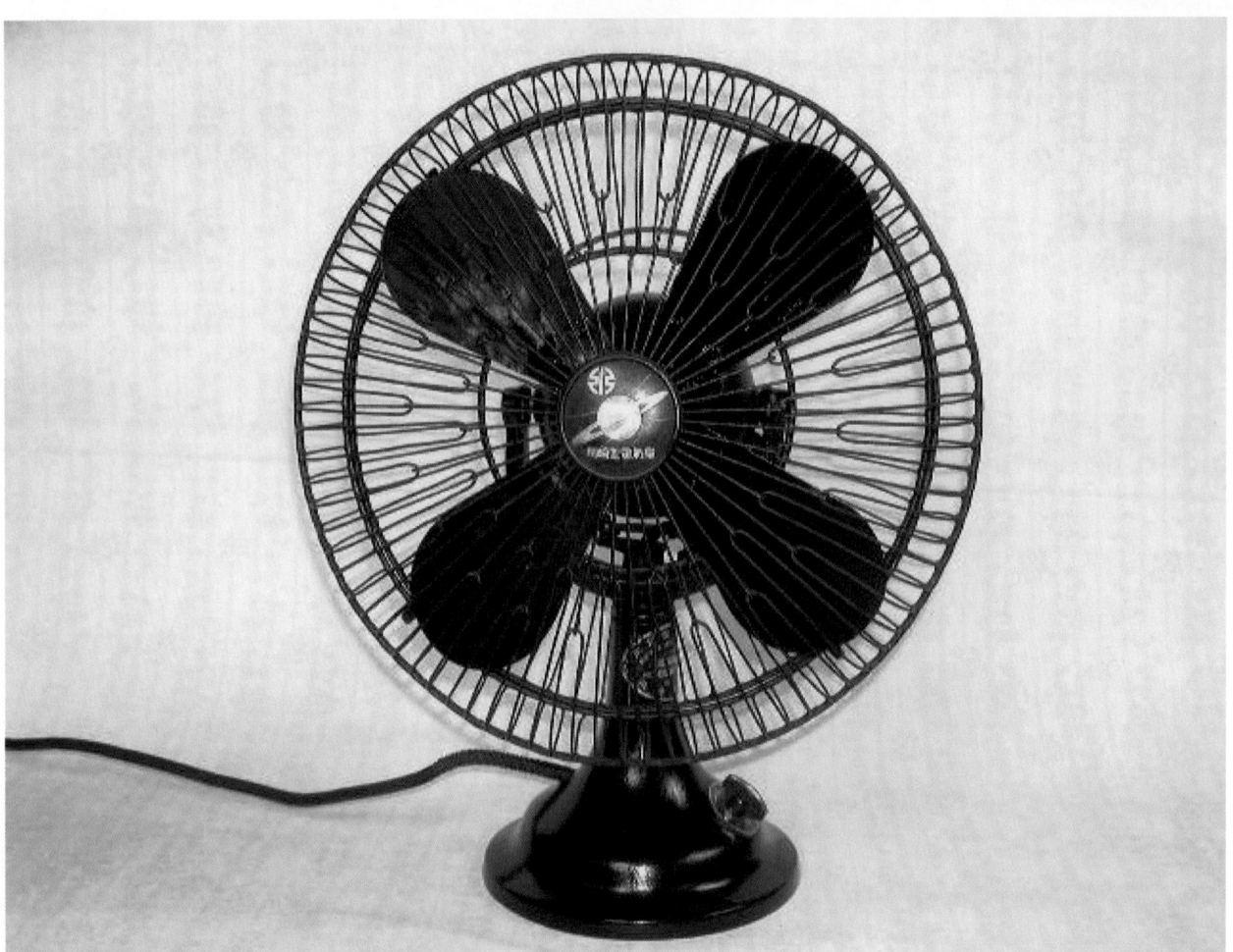

1. I'm hot. Turn on the _____.

2. What does it do?

3. When do you use it?

4. Where do you keep it?

5. Make a sound like a fan.

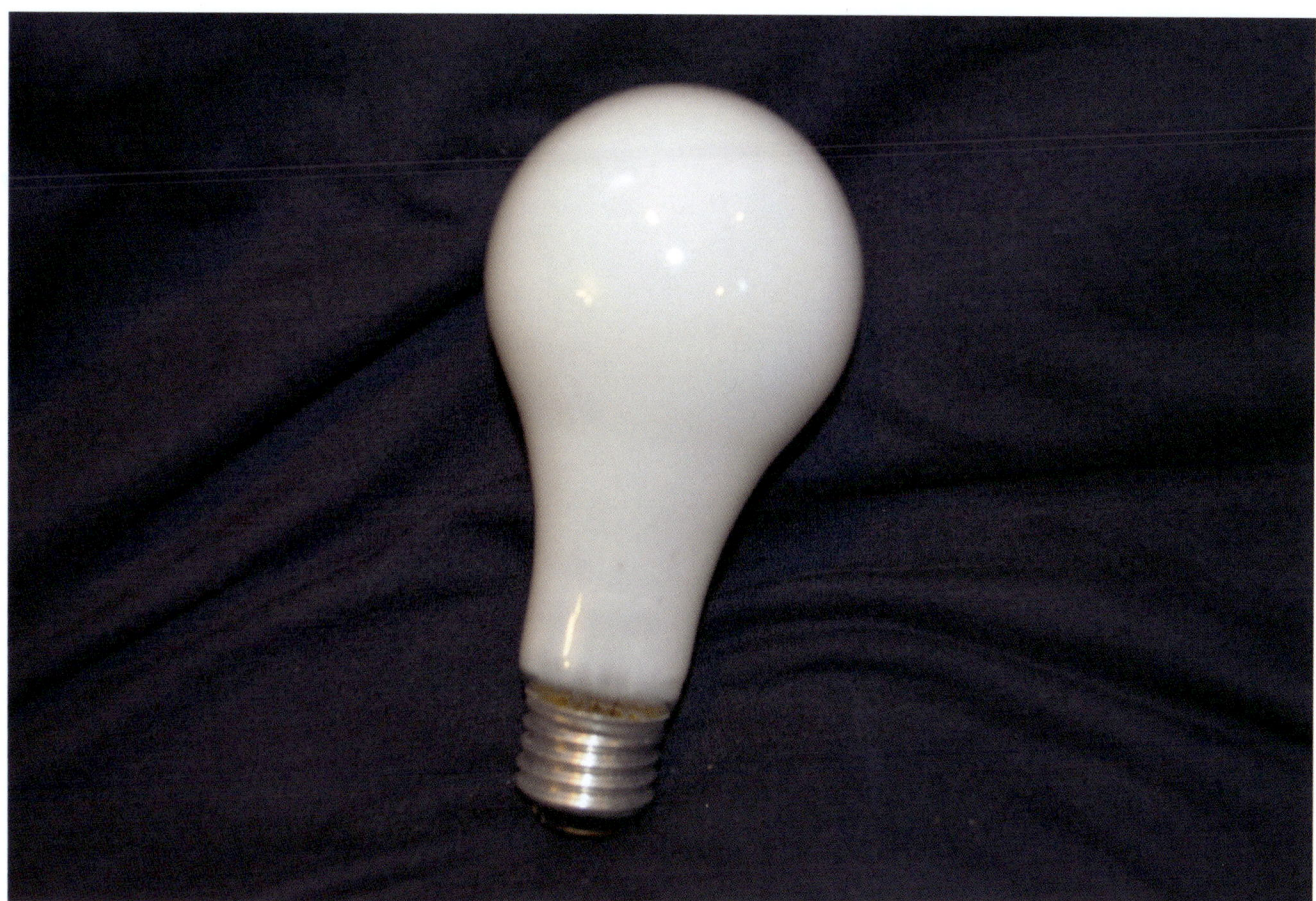

xliii

1. It is time to change the light _____.

2. Where does it go?

3. What does it do?

4. How does it work?

5. Pretend you are screwing one in.

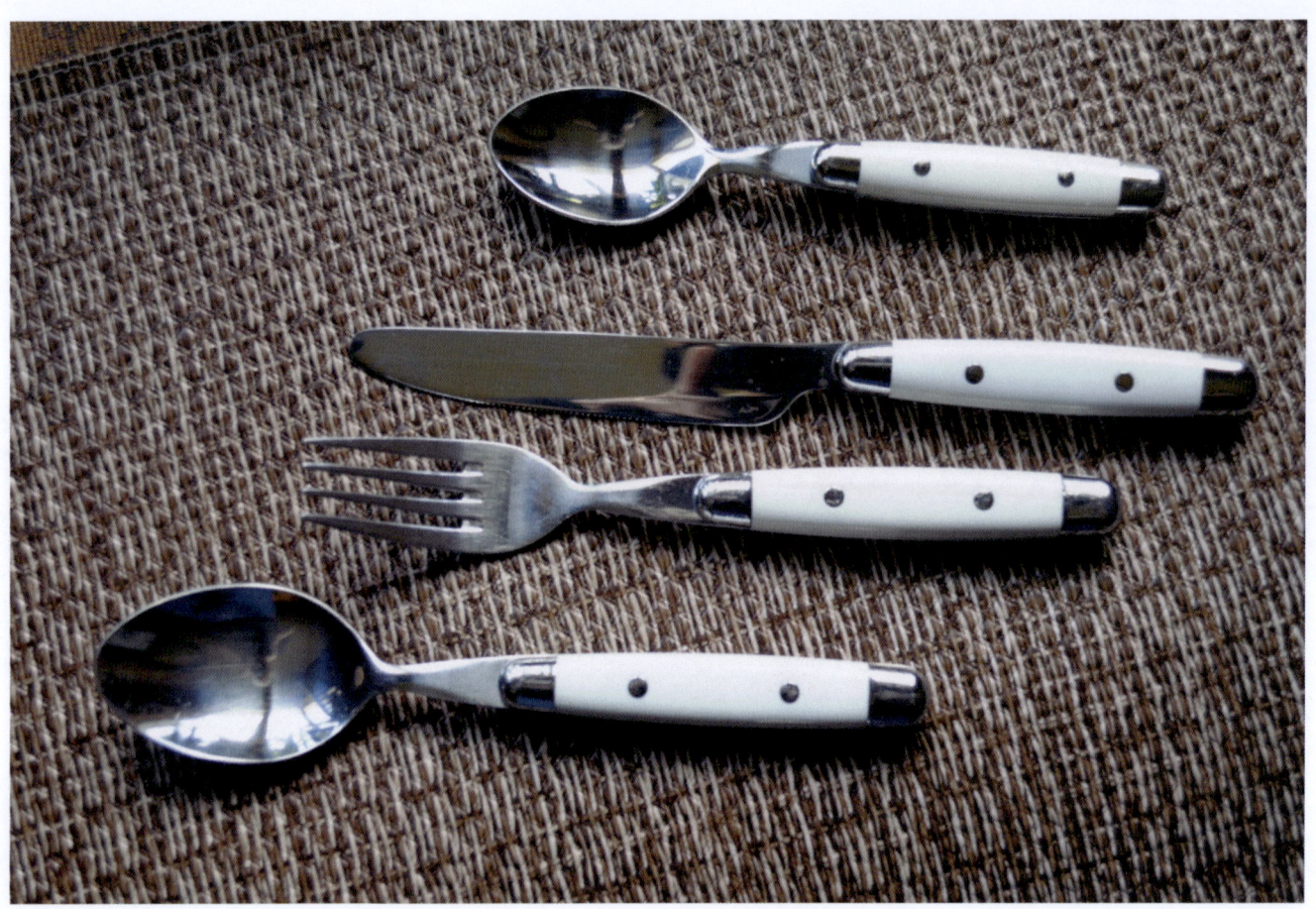

xliv

1.   Set the table with the _____.

2.   Where do you keep them?

3.   Describe where they go around a plate.

4.   What two types of spoons are there?

5.   Pretend you are cutting meat with a knife.

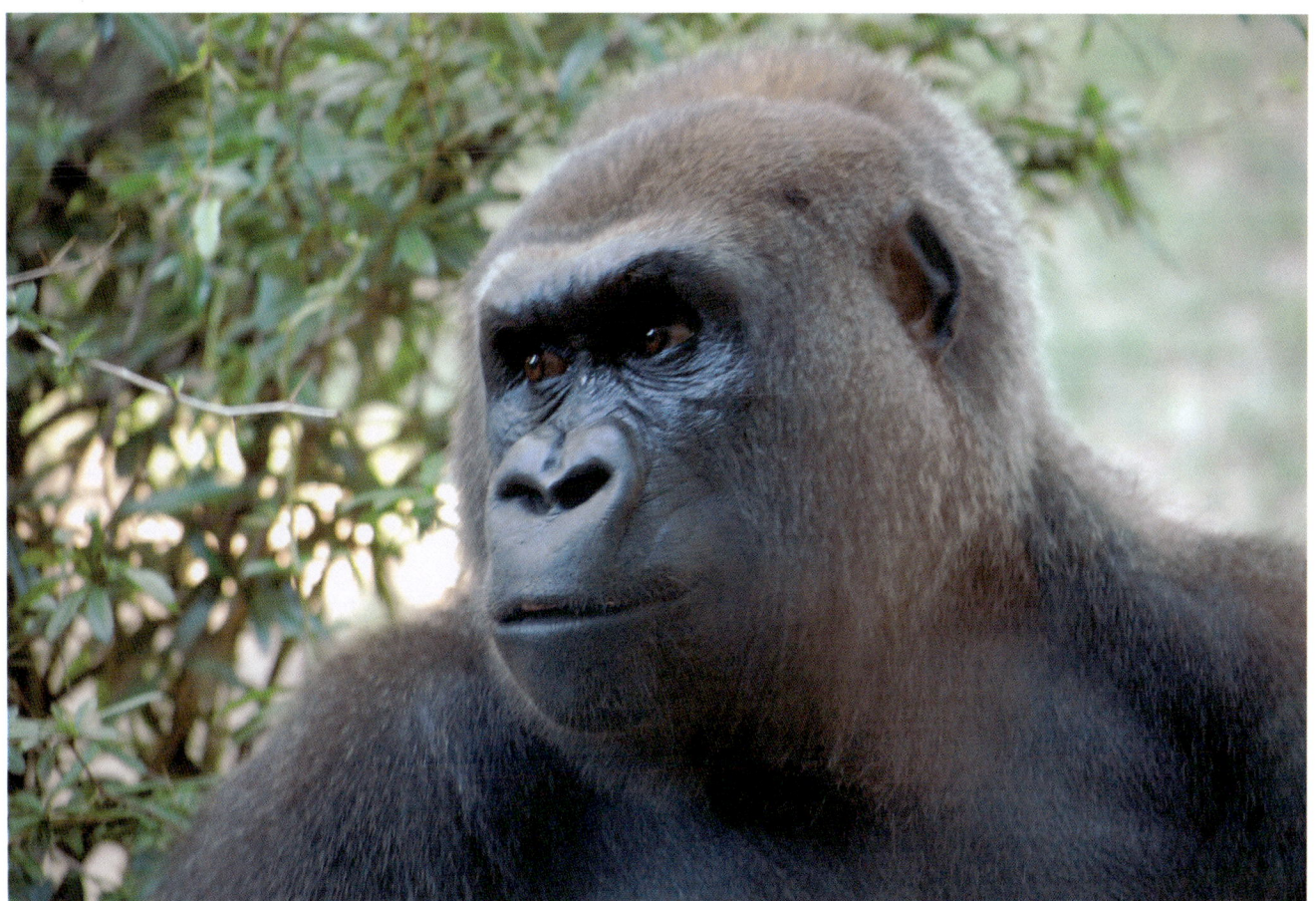

1. I went to the zoo and saw a _____.

2. Where do they live in the wild?

3. What color is its fur?

4. Can you name a famous anthropologist who studied them?

5. Make a sound and gesture like one.

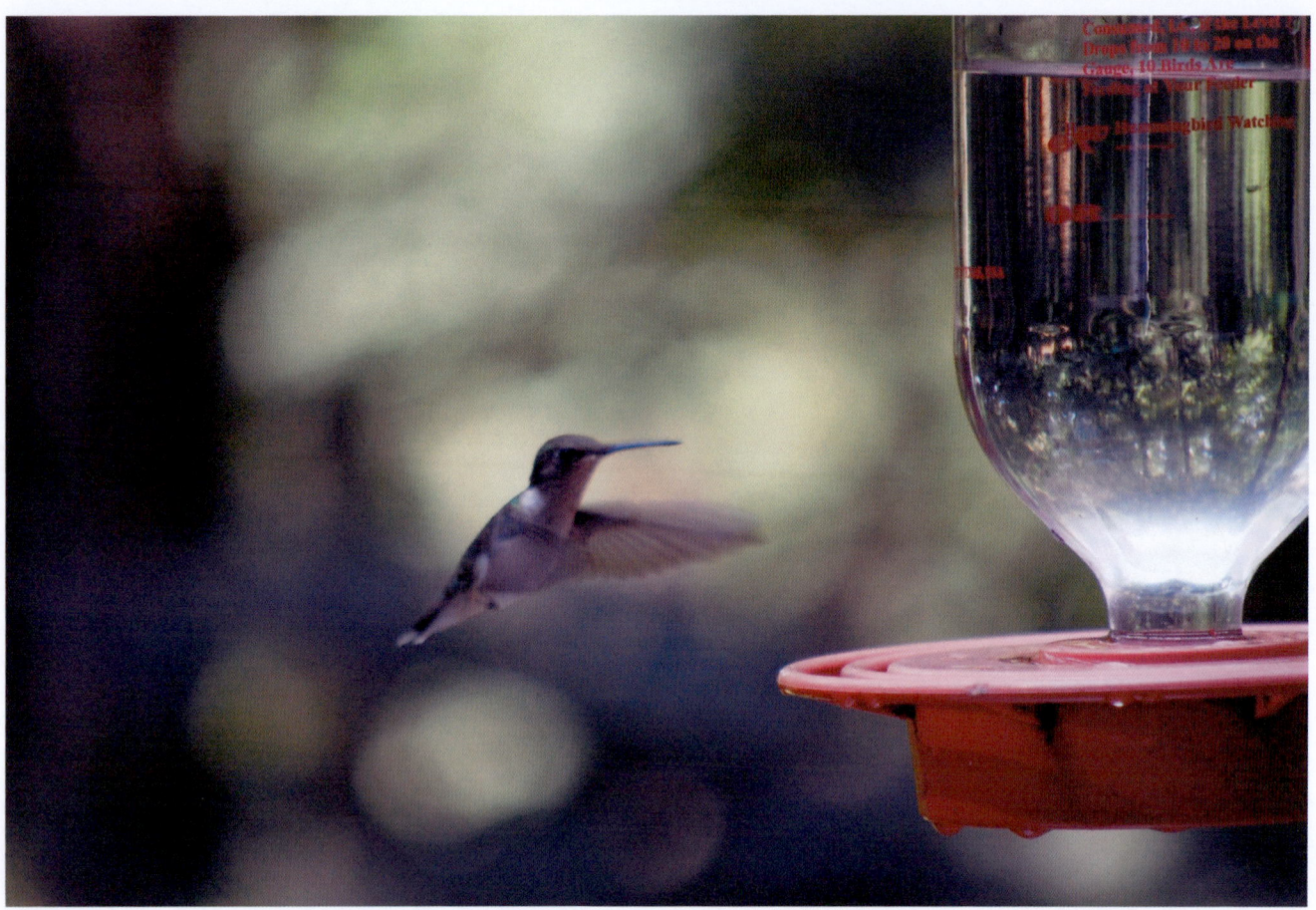

xlvi

1.   Look at that tiny little _____.

2.   What do they eat?

3.   How big are they?

4.   Where do they live?

5.   Make a sound like one.

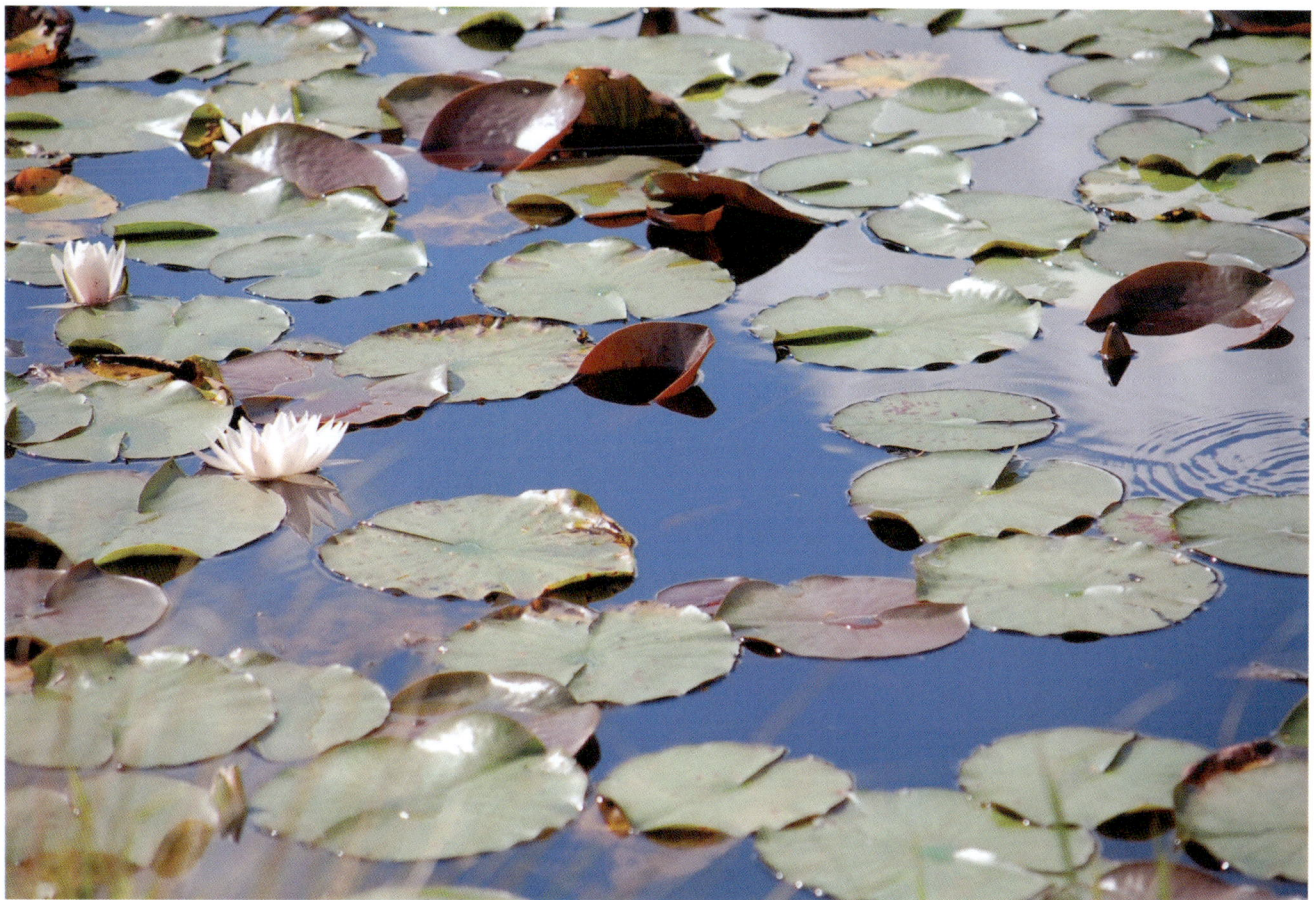

xlvii

1.　The frog jumped on the lily _____.

2.　Where do you find them?

3.　What color are they?

4.　Do they float or sink?

5.　What shape are they?

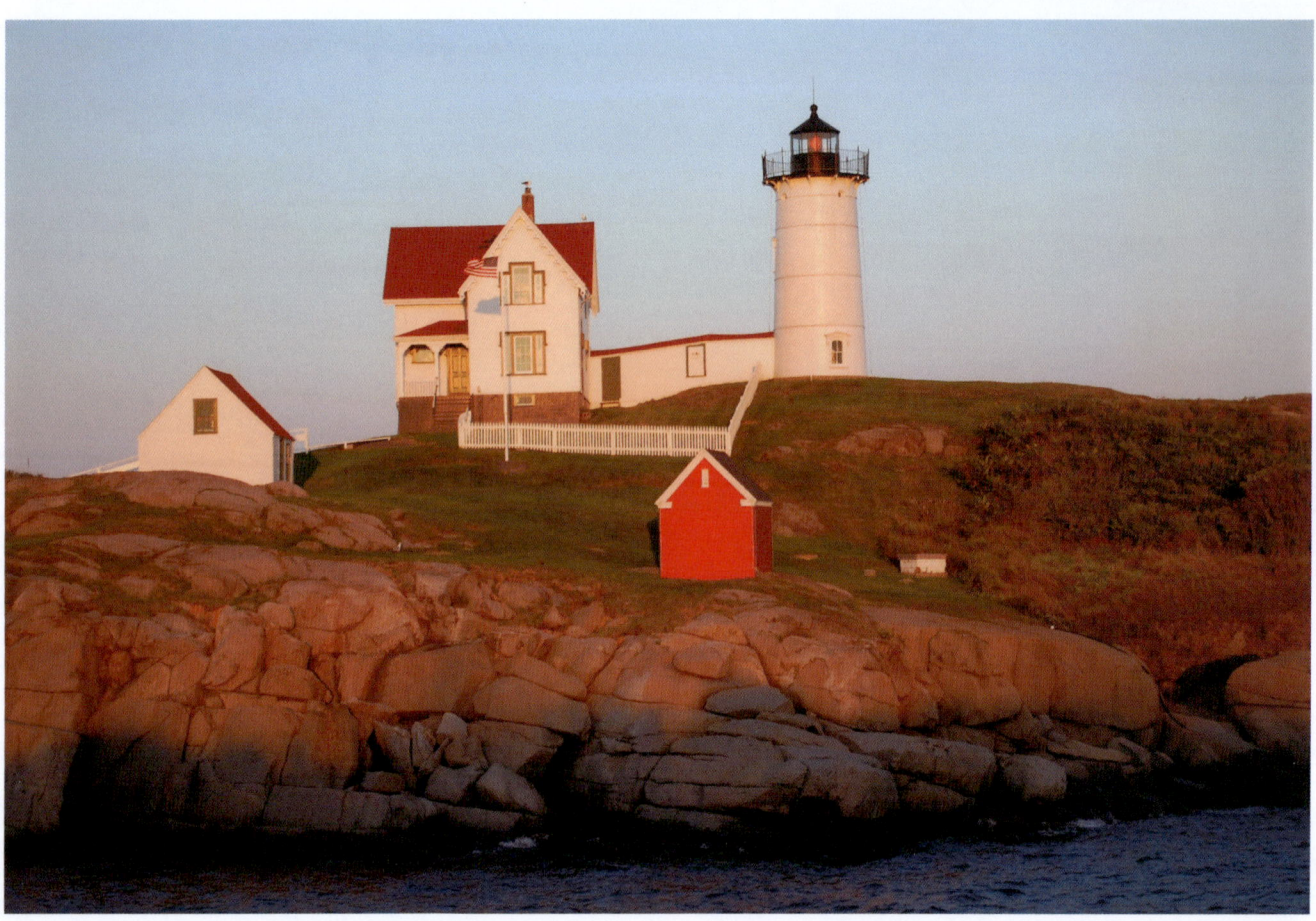

1.   The boat saw the light from the light _____.

2.   Where would you find one?

3.   What are they for?

4.   Have you ever seen one?

5.   Where do you think this one is located?

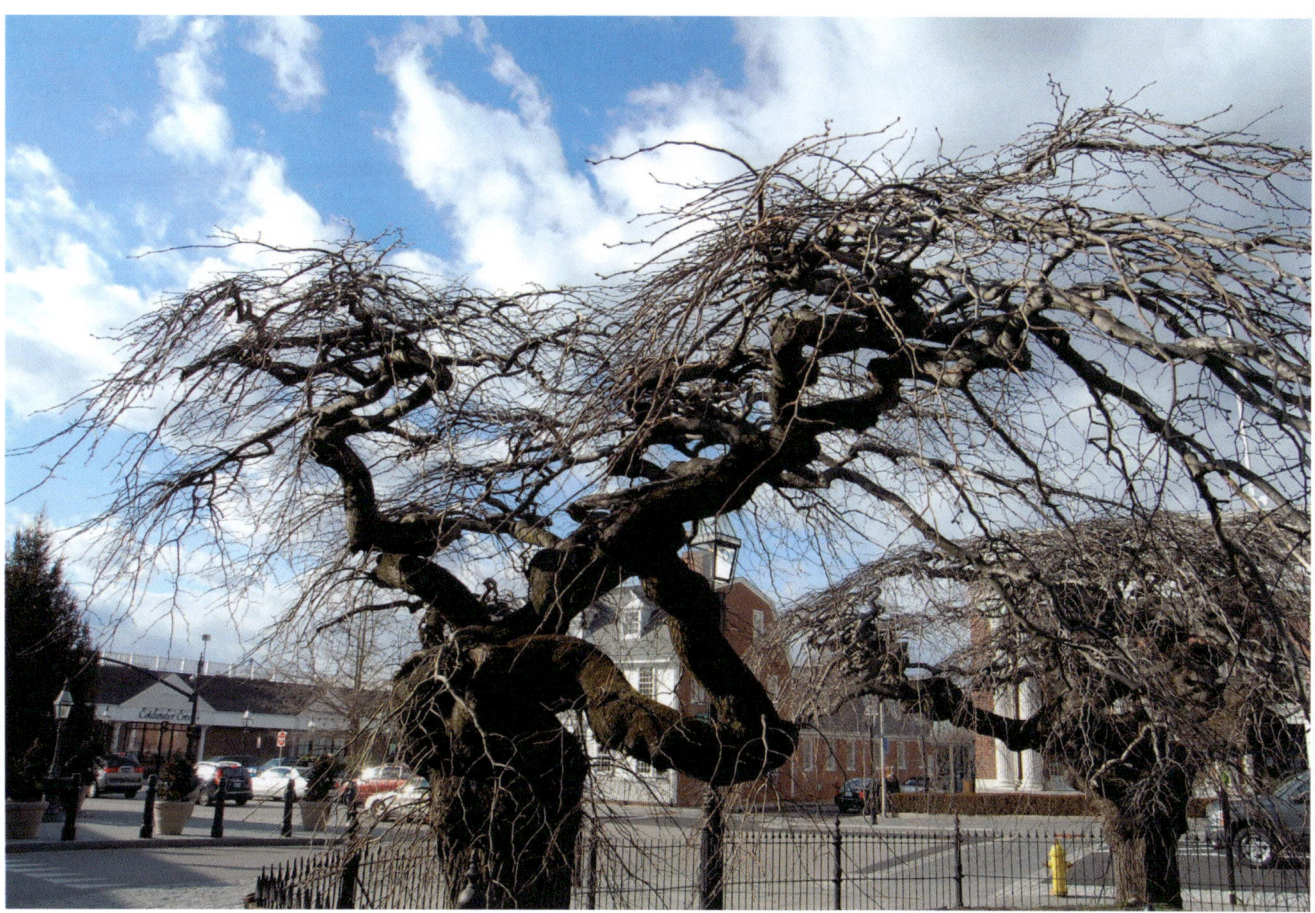

xlix

1. I'd like the climb that_____.

2. What time of year is it?

3. Where is it located?

4. What is unique about this tree?

5. What is it missing?

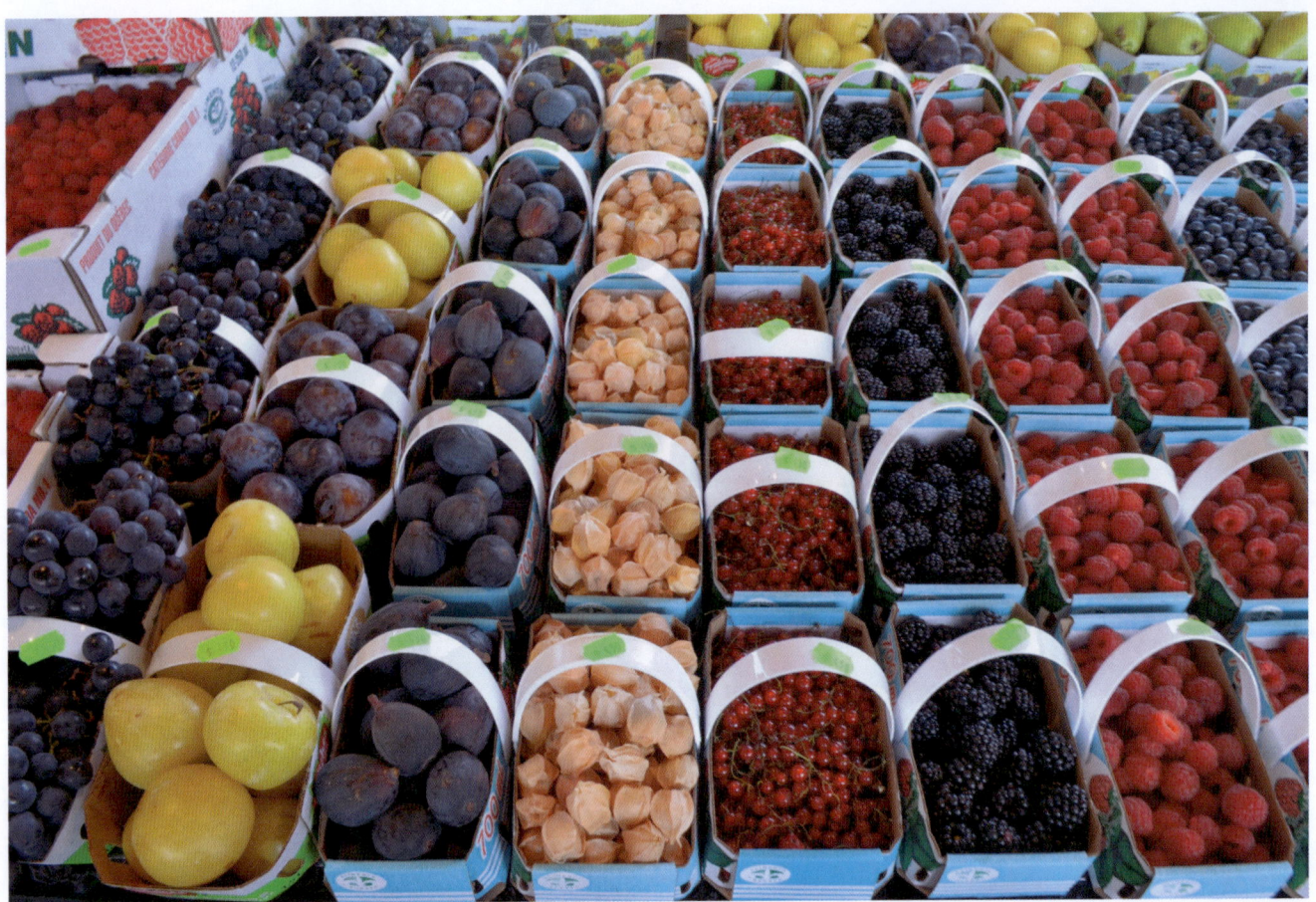

1. Wow look at all the fresh _____.

2. What containers are they in?

3. Name three types of berries that are in the photo.

4. What color are the grapes in the photo?

5. Which basket would you like to have?

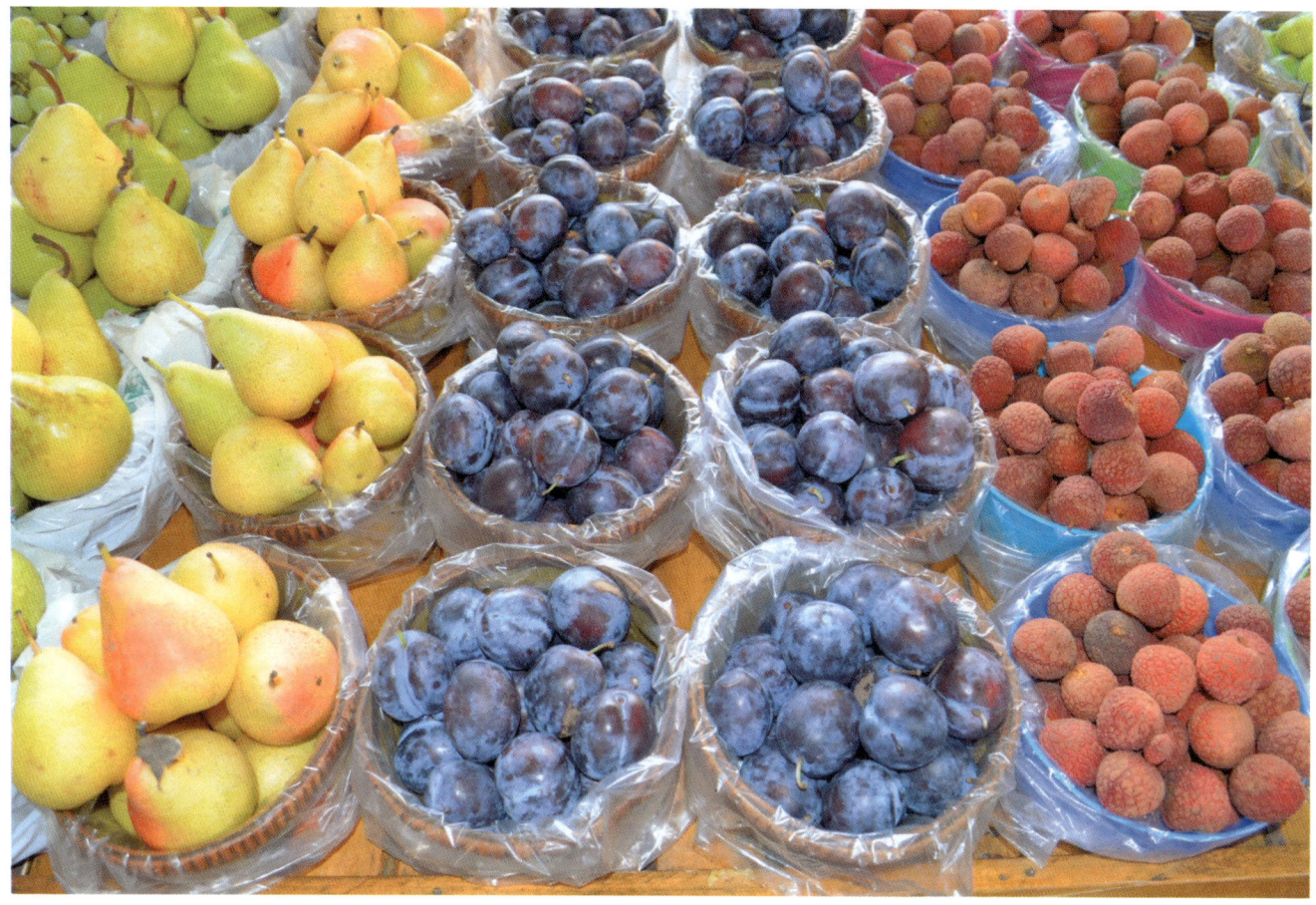

li

1. I'm going to buy a large basket of _____.

2. What colors are the fruit?

3. Which fruit is blue?

4. Which fruit is yellow and green?

5. Which one is your favorite?

Famous Places and Things

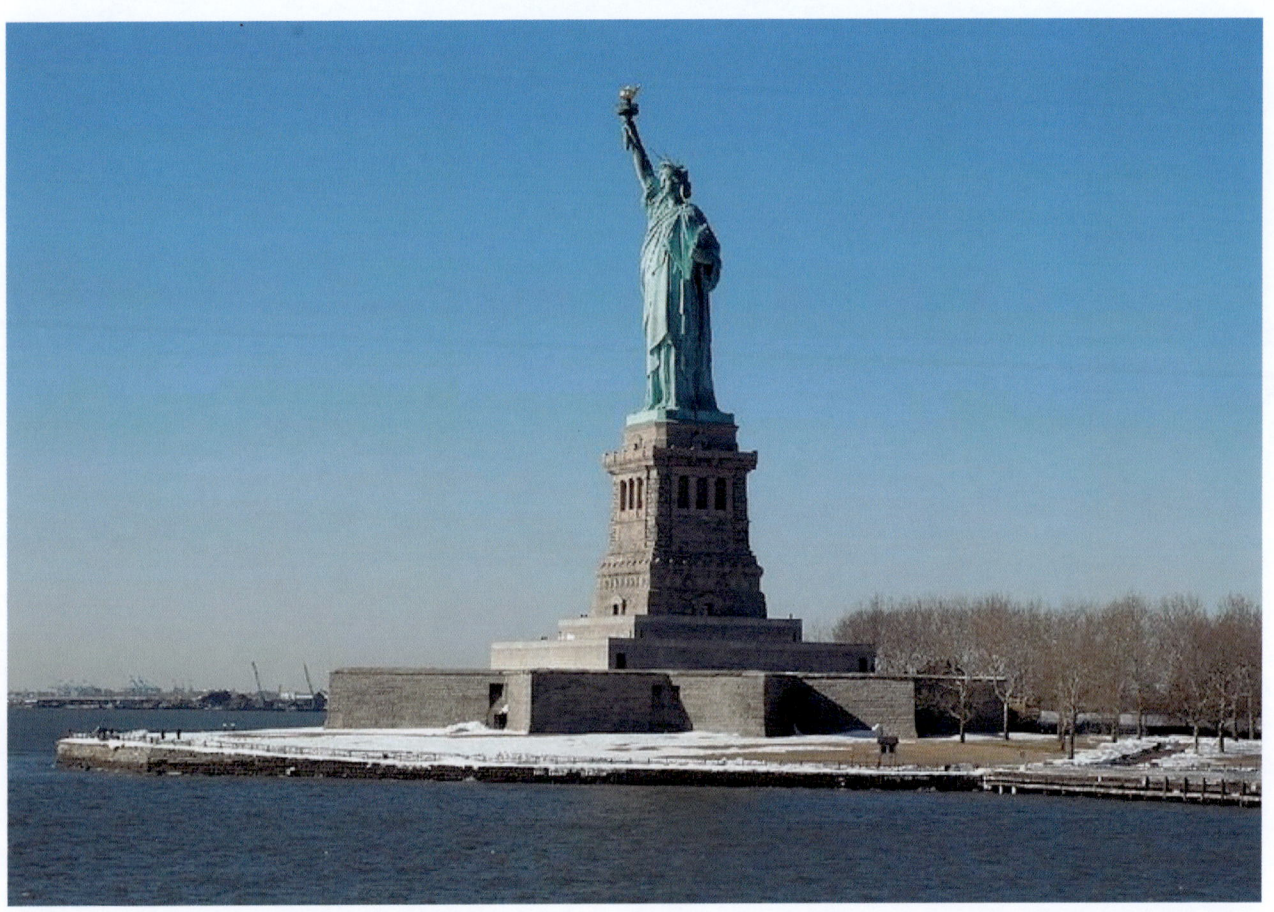

lii

1.   I've always wanted to see the _____.

2.   Where is it?

3.   What does it stand for?

4.   What can you do if you visit it?

5.   Pretend you are the statue.

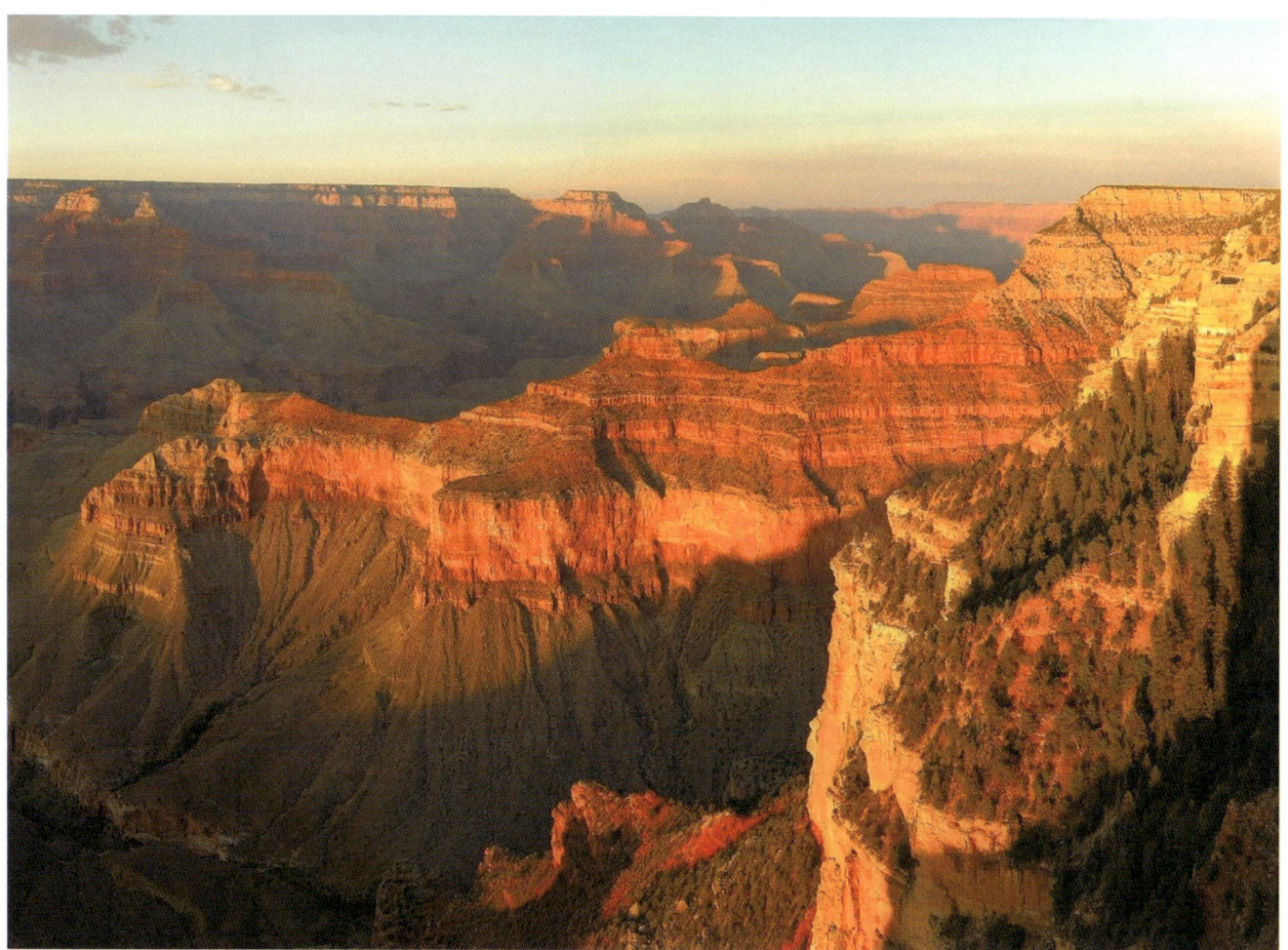

liii

1. I'm going hiking in the Grand _____.

2. Where is it?

3. What can people do there?

4. Have you ever been there?

5. Describe the photograph.

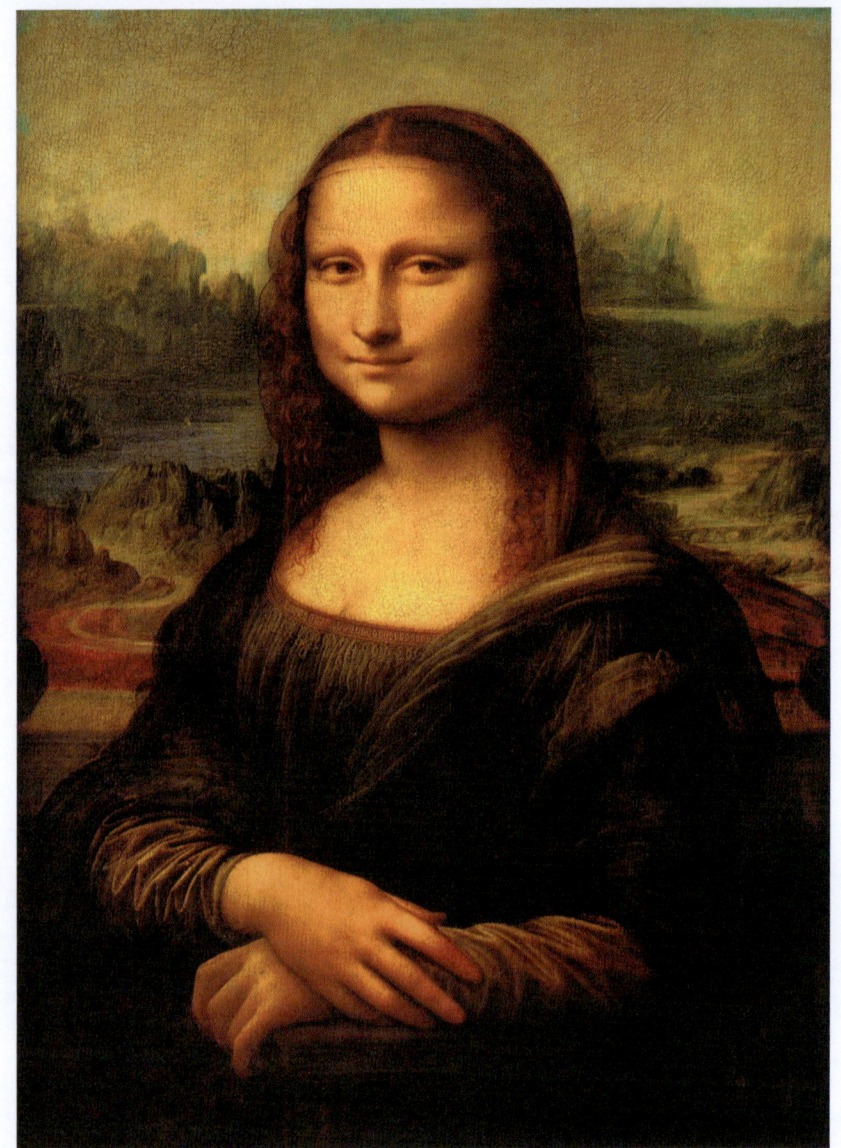

liv

1.   Leonardo Da Vinci painted the _____.

2.   What is she doing?

3.   Where is the painting located?

4.   How much do you think the painting is worth?

5.   Have you ever seen it?

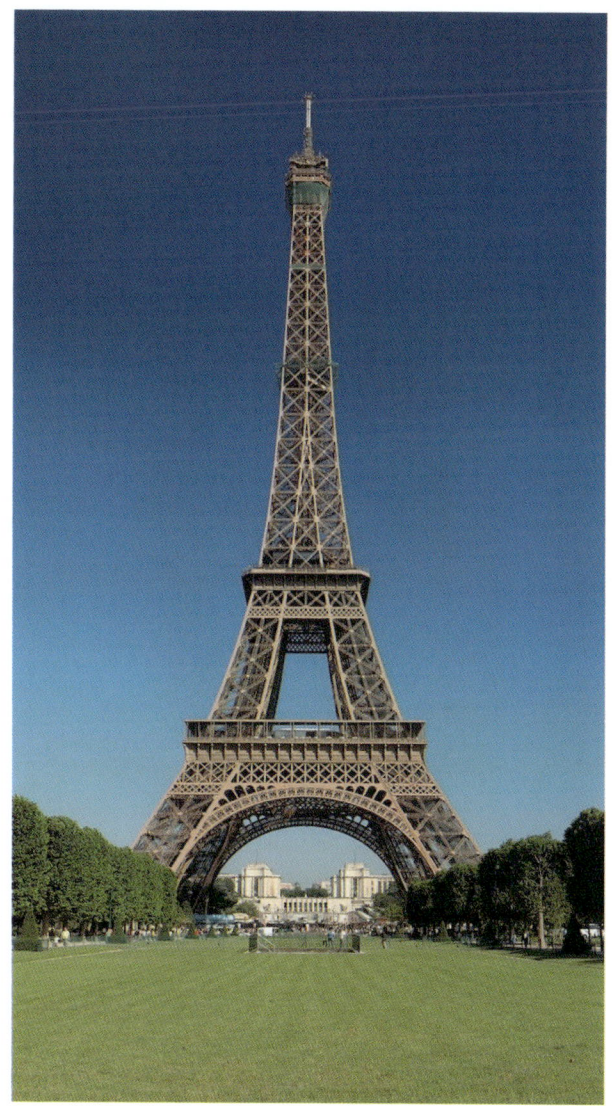

lv

1.   Lets go to the top of the _____.

2.   What country is it in?

3.   What city is it in?

4.   Have you ever seen it?

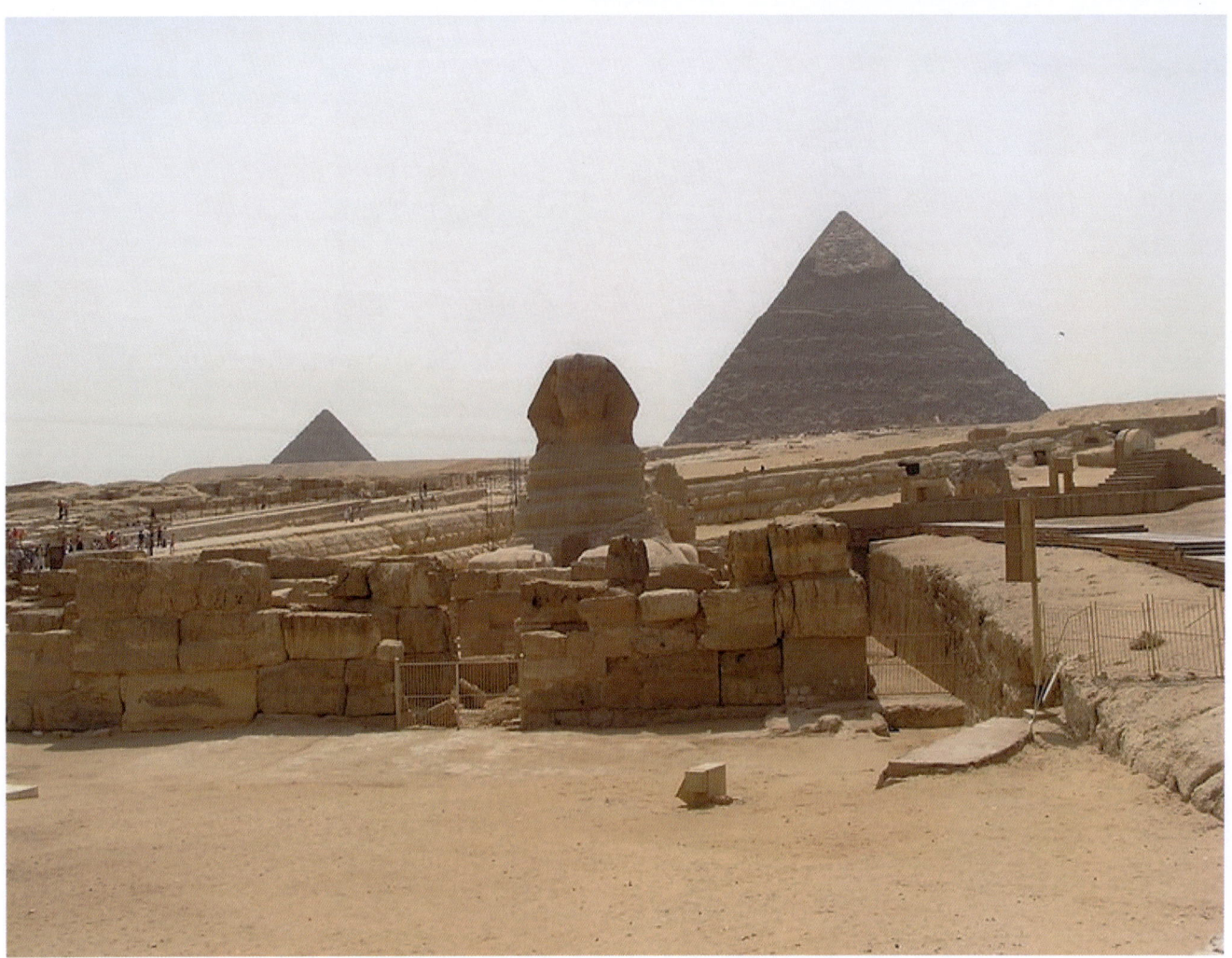

lvi

1. I'm excited to see the ancient _____.

2. Where are they?

3. Around when were they built?

4. Who is buried inside them?

5. Have you ever seen them?

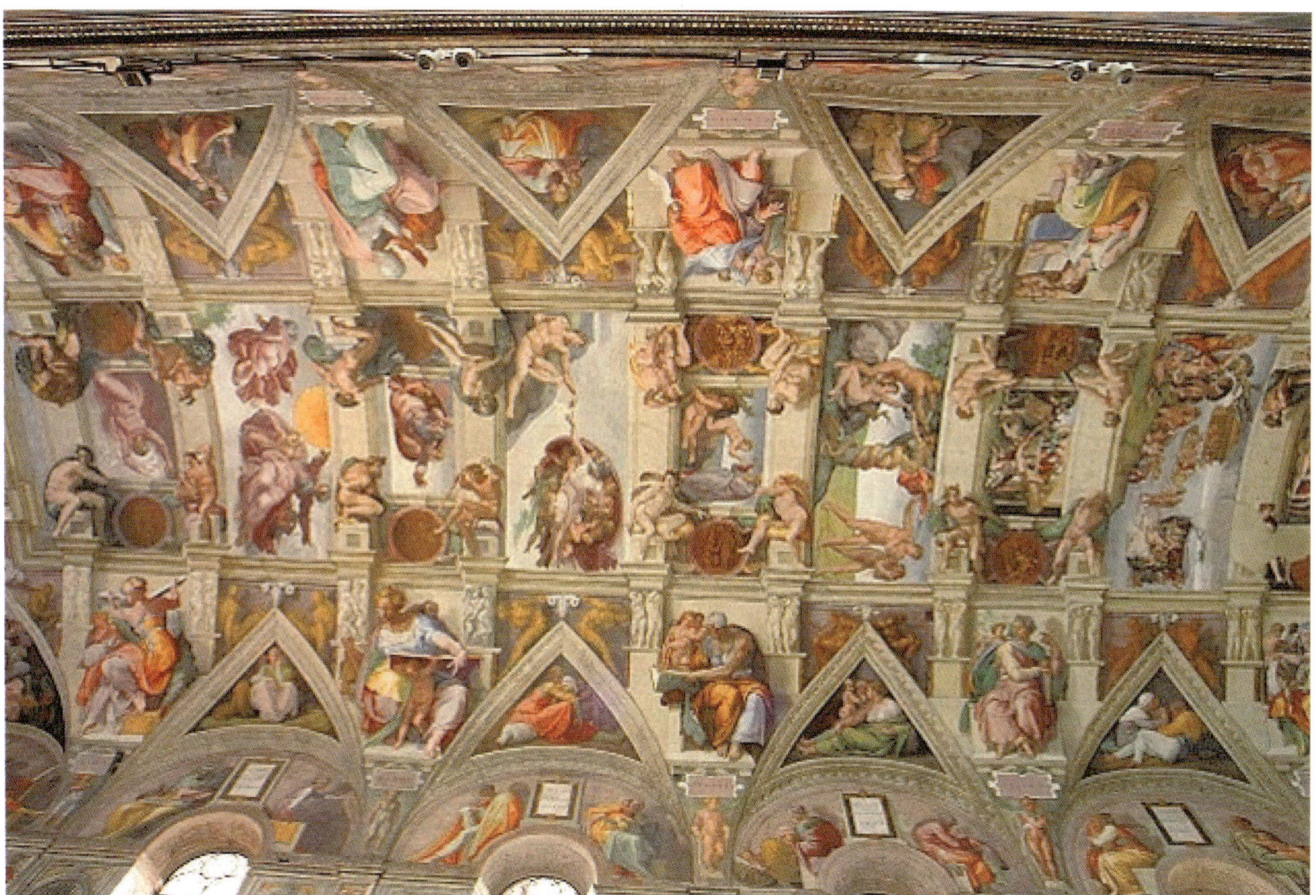

lvii

1.   Michelangelo painted a masterpiece on the ceiling of the _____.

2.   Where is it?

3.   Have you ever seen it?

4.   What does it depict?

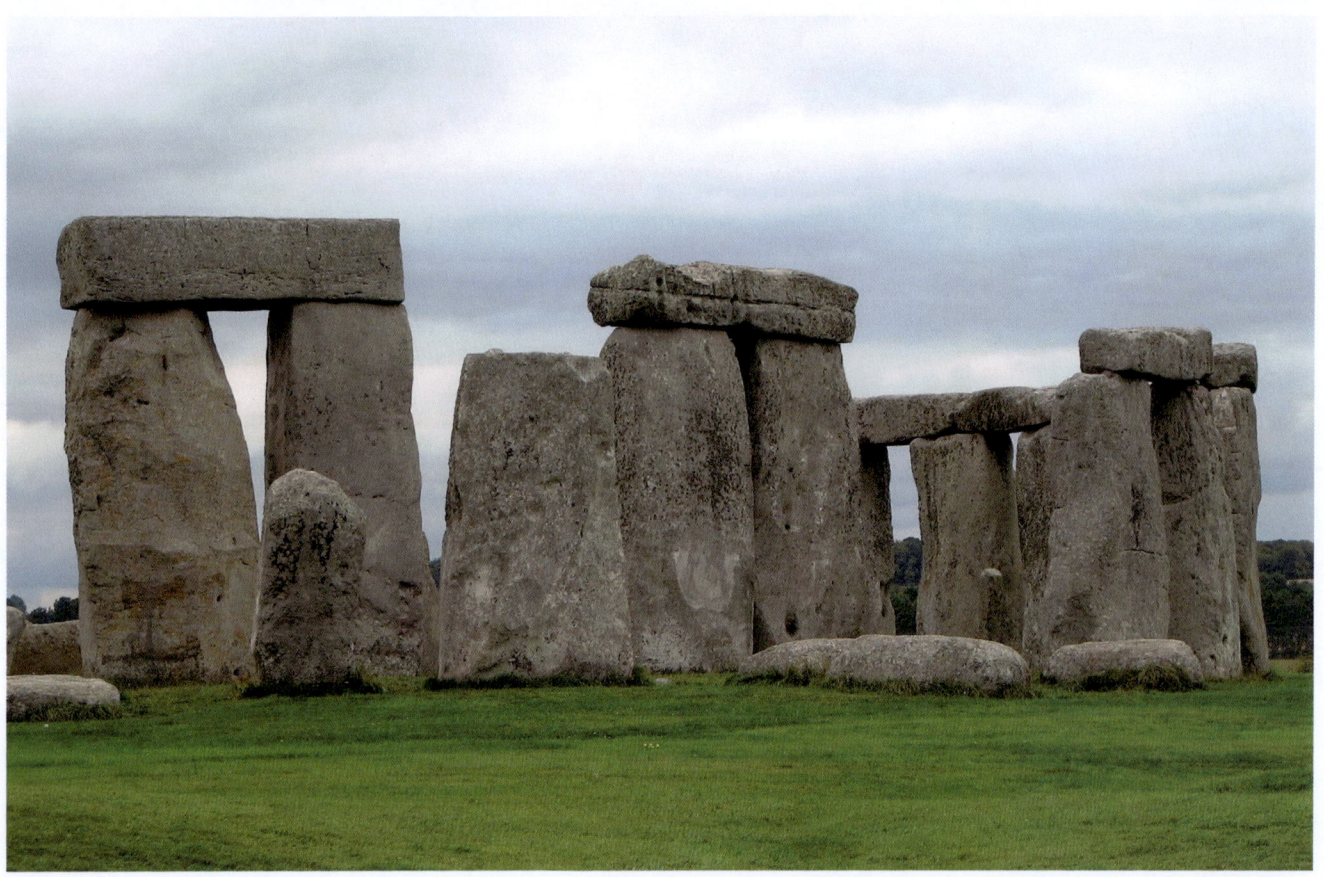

lviii

1. On my vacation, I took a lot of pictures of _____.

2. Where is it?

3. What is it?

4. About how old do you think it is?

5. Have you ever seen it?

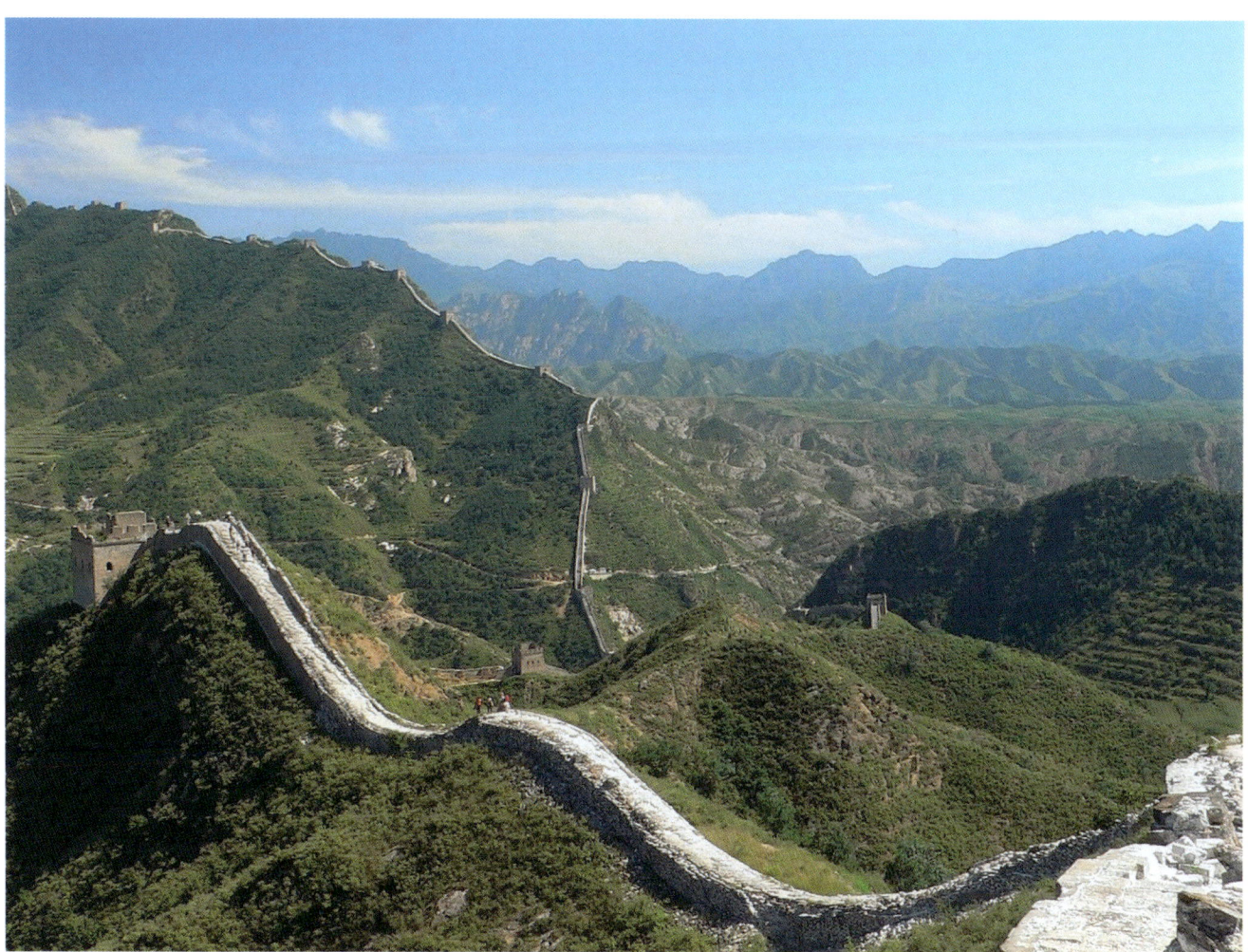

lix

1.   The only man made object visible from space is the _____.

2.   Where is it?

3.   Why was it built?

4.   About how long ago was it built?

5.   Have you ever seen it?

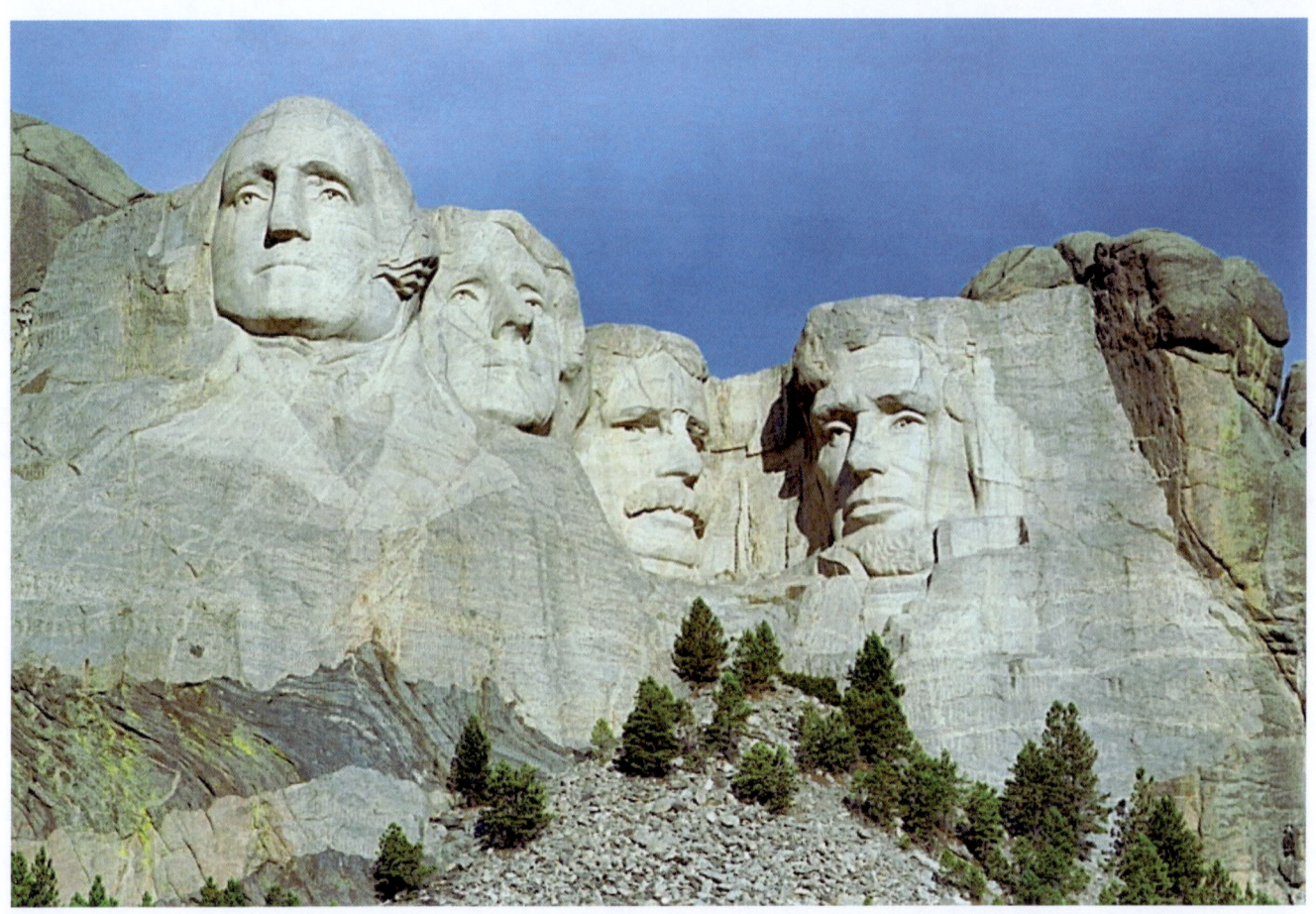

lx

1. I am planning a vacation to see Mt. _____.

2. Who is on the mountainside?

3. Name two of the presidents.

4. Have you ever been there?

66

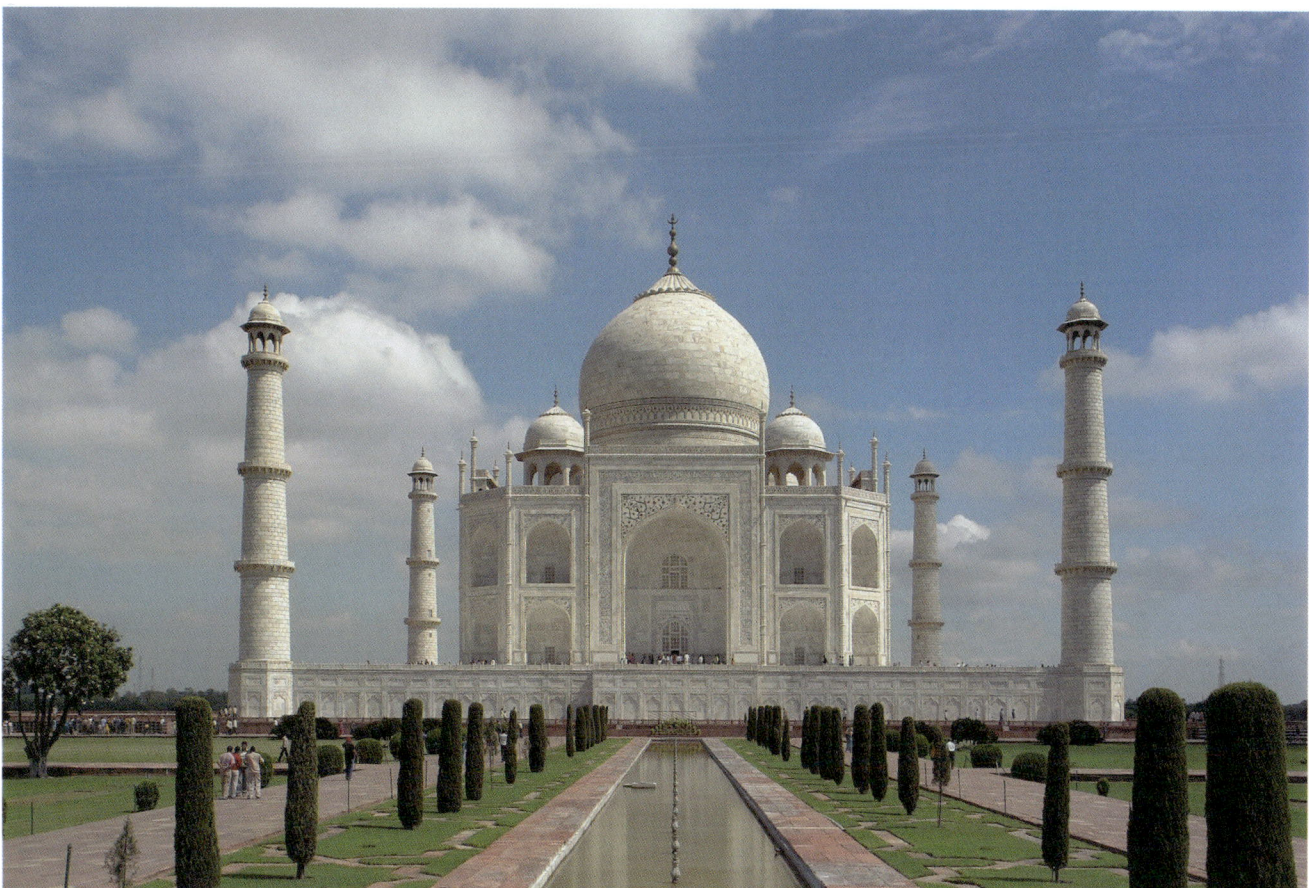

lxi

1. I've never been to see the _____.

2. What is it?

3. Where is it located?

4. Have you ever been there?

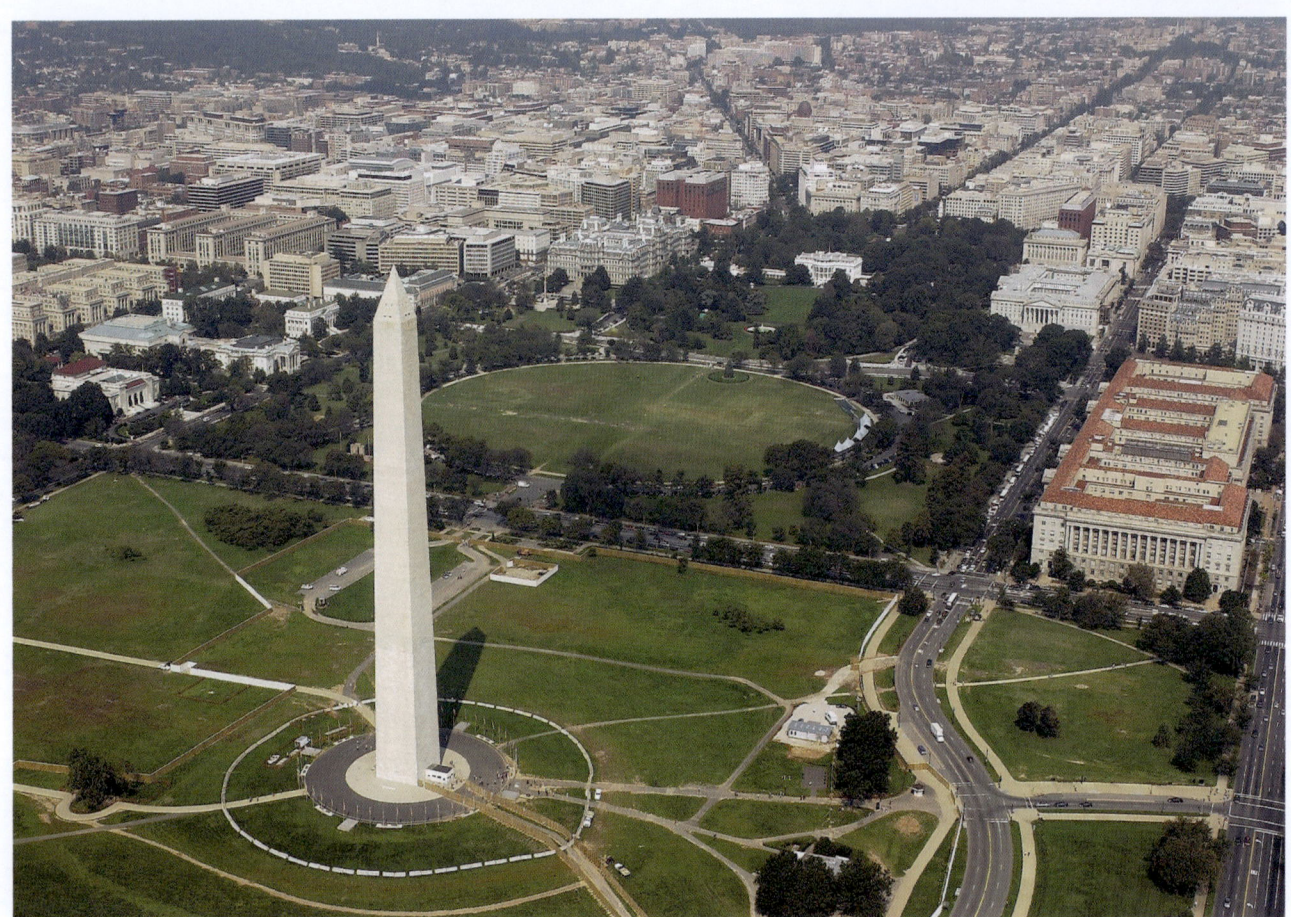

lxii

1.	That is an aerial view of the _____.

2.	What city is it in?

3.	Have you ever seen it?

4.	Have you ever been inside it?

5.	What other famous buildings are on the National Mall?

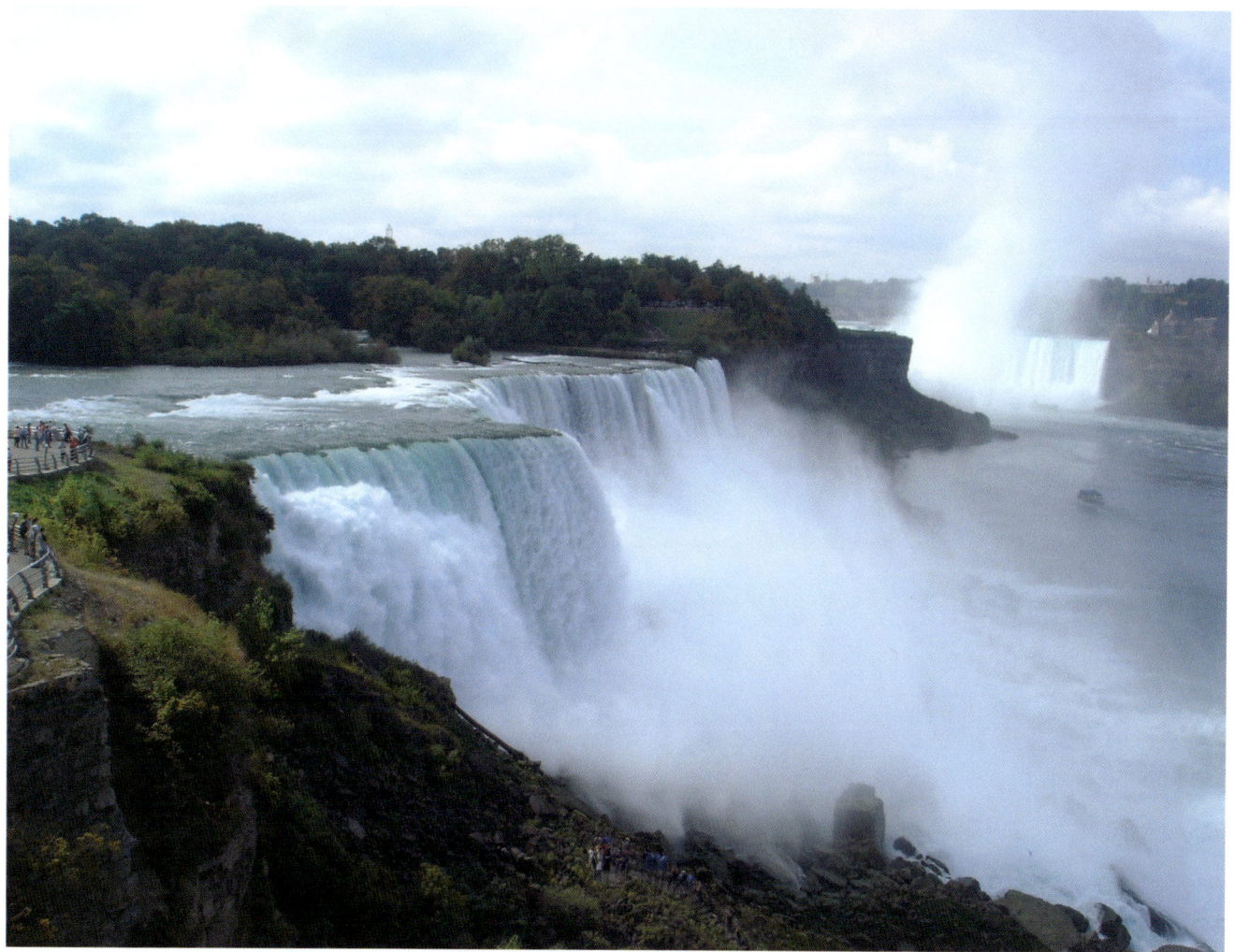

lxiii

1. The view is breathtaking at Niagara _____.

2. What two countries border the falls?

3. Explain what is needed in order to have a waterfall.

4. Have you ever been there? If so, describe your trip.

5. What other recreational activities are available at Niagara Falls?

Of all the photos of famous places which one would you like to see the most?

Safety Awareness

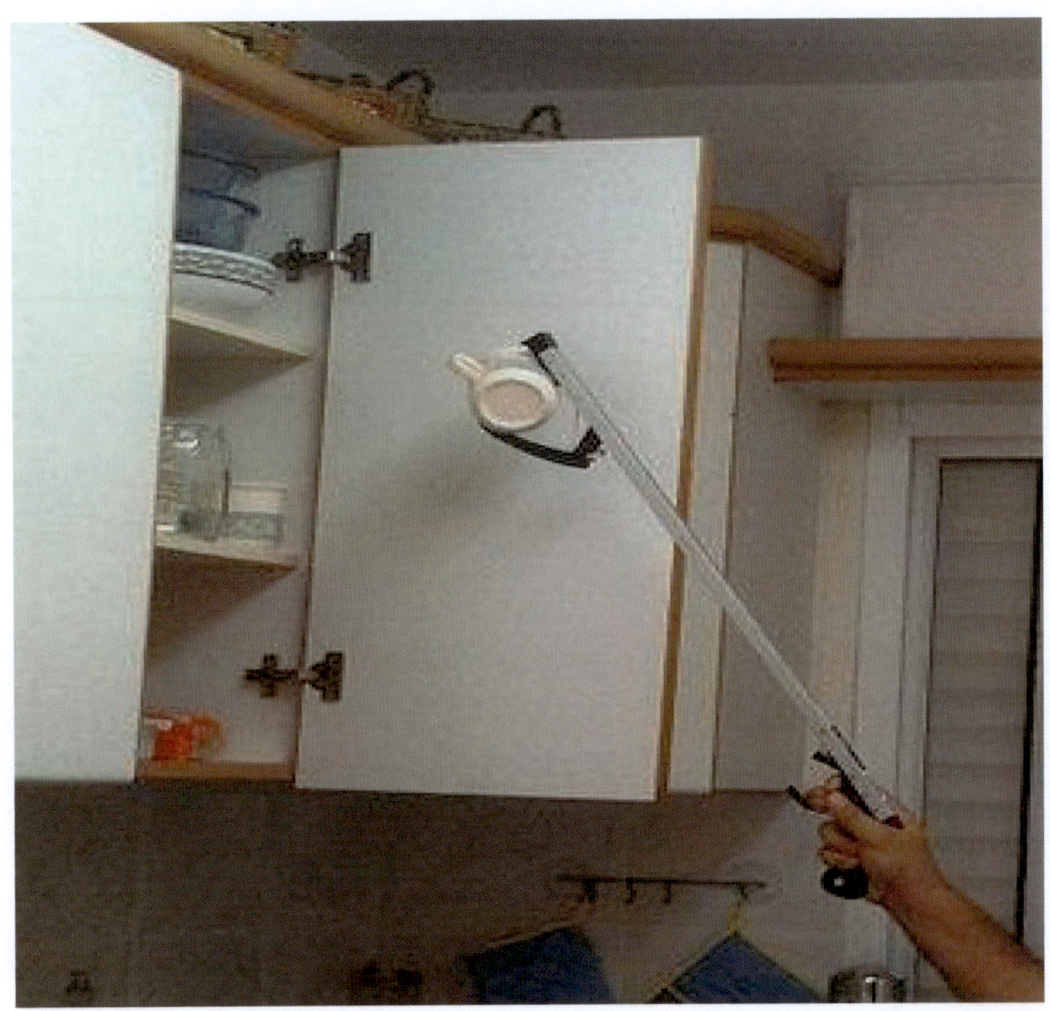

lxiv

1. He was able to get his coffee cup with a _____.

2. Why is a reacher a safer alternative?

3. What could happen if somebody with limited strength didn't use a reacher?

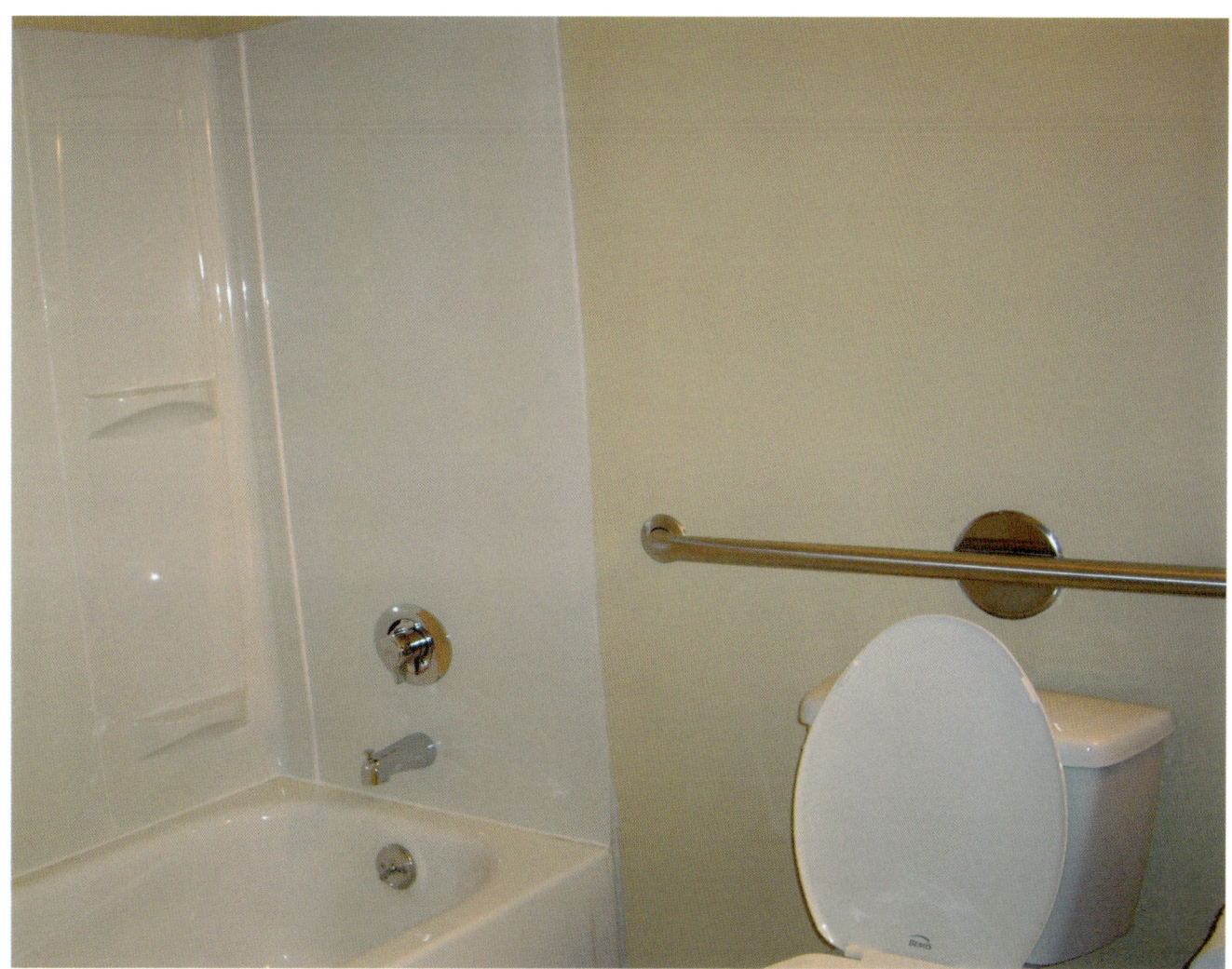

lxv

1.   What safety device is installed in this bathroom?

2.   Why should somebody use it?

3.   What else can they install to make the bathroom safer?

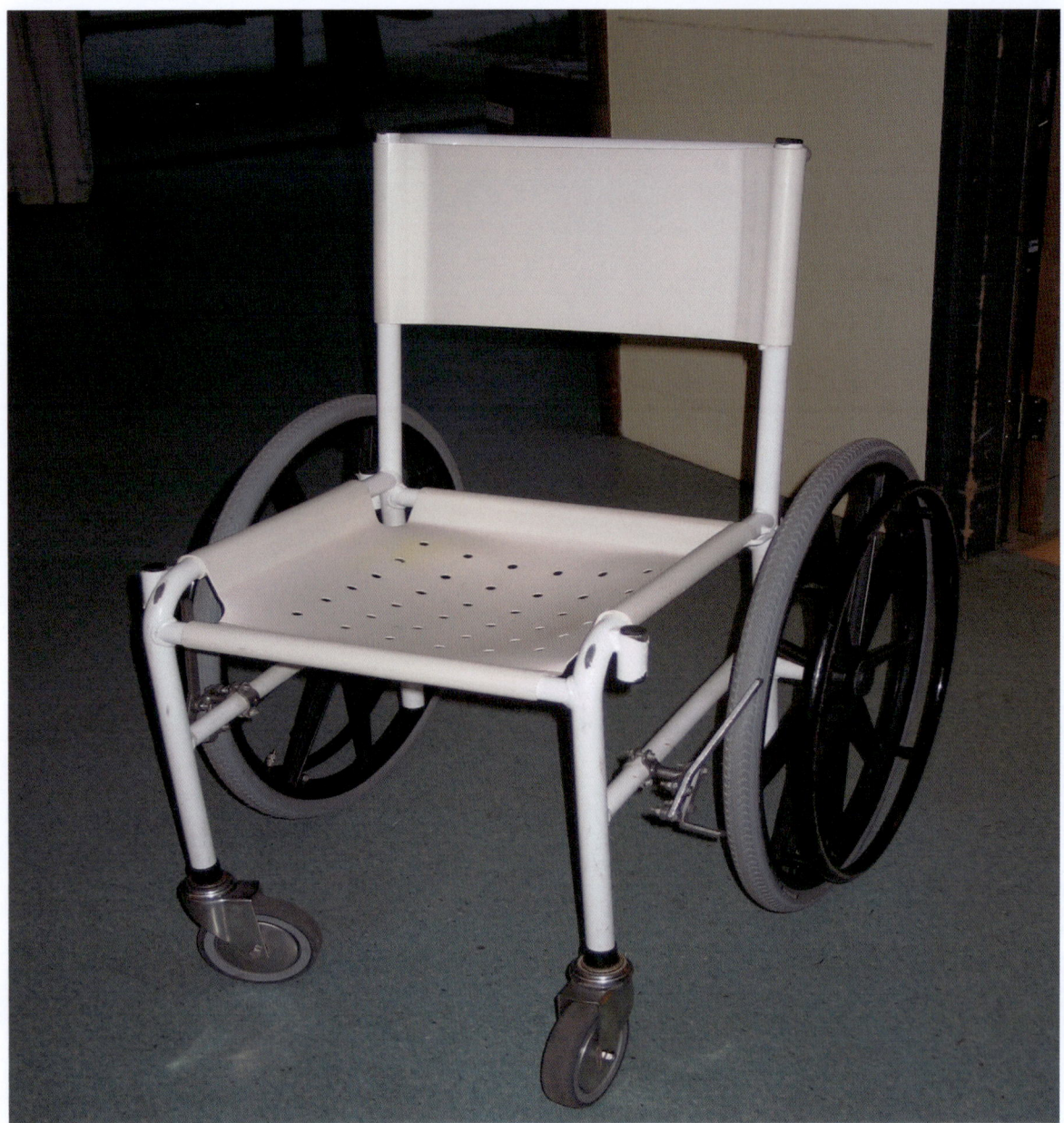

lxvi

1. Why would a shower chair be helpful?

2. What must always be locked on the wheelchair before somebody stands up?

3. Describe how somebody could use this safety device.

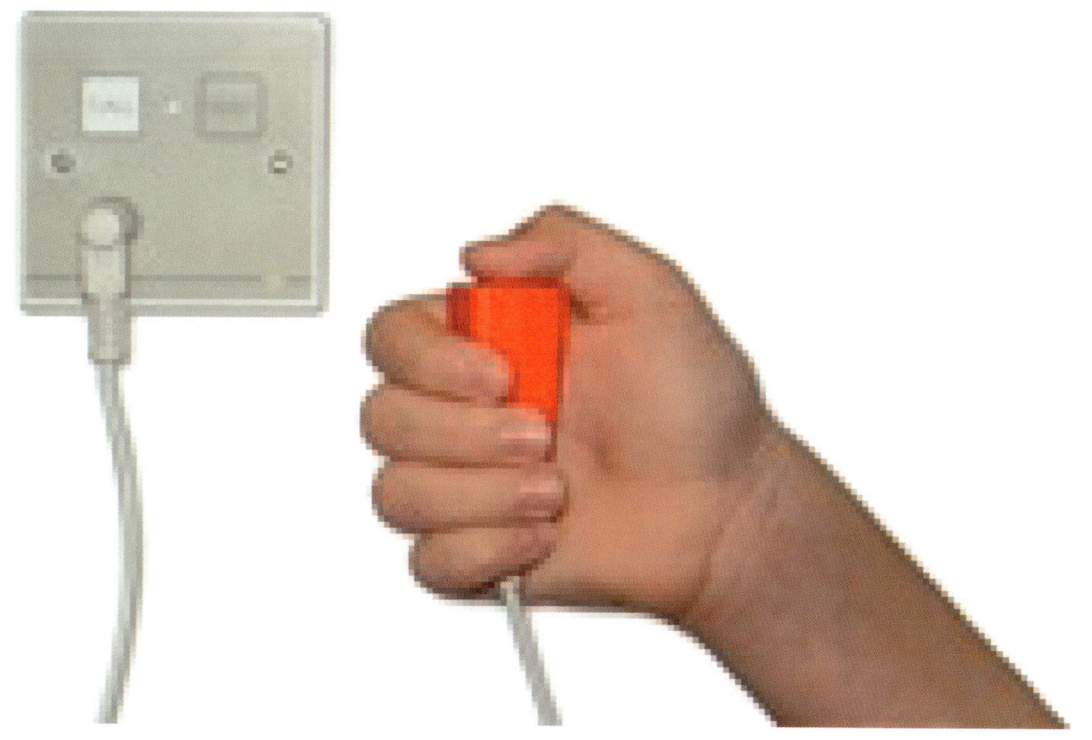

lxvii

1. I need help! I should push my _____.

2. What does it do?

3. When should you use it?

4. Where can you find one?

5. Do you have one?

73

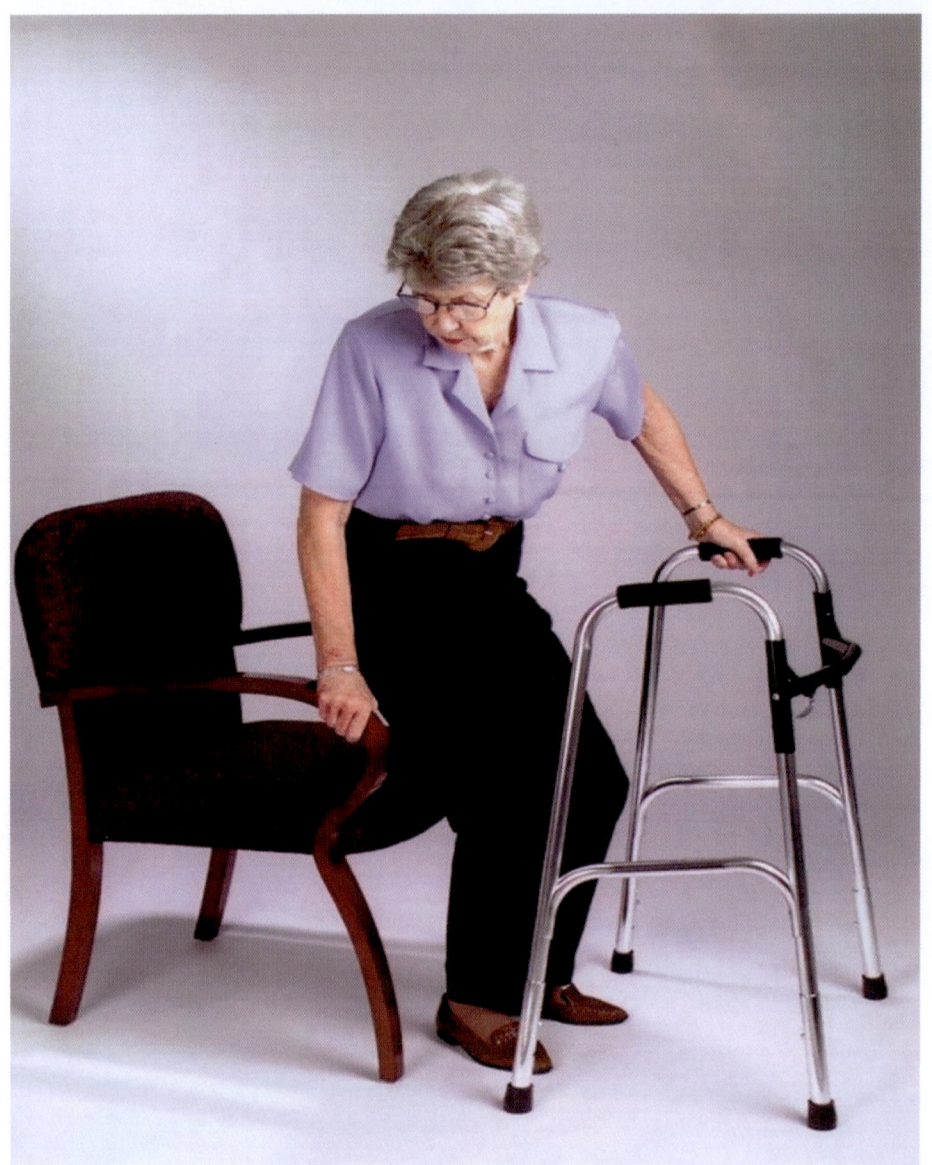

1. What is she doing?

2. Explain how she is sitting down safely.

3. What should you always do before you sit down?

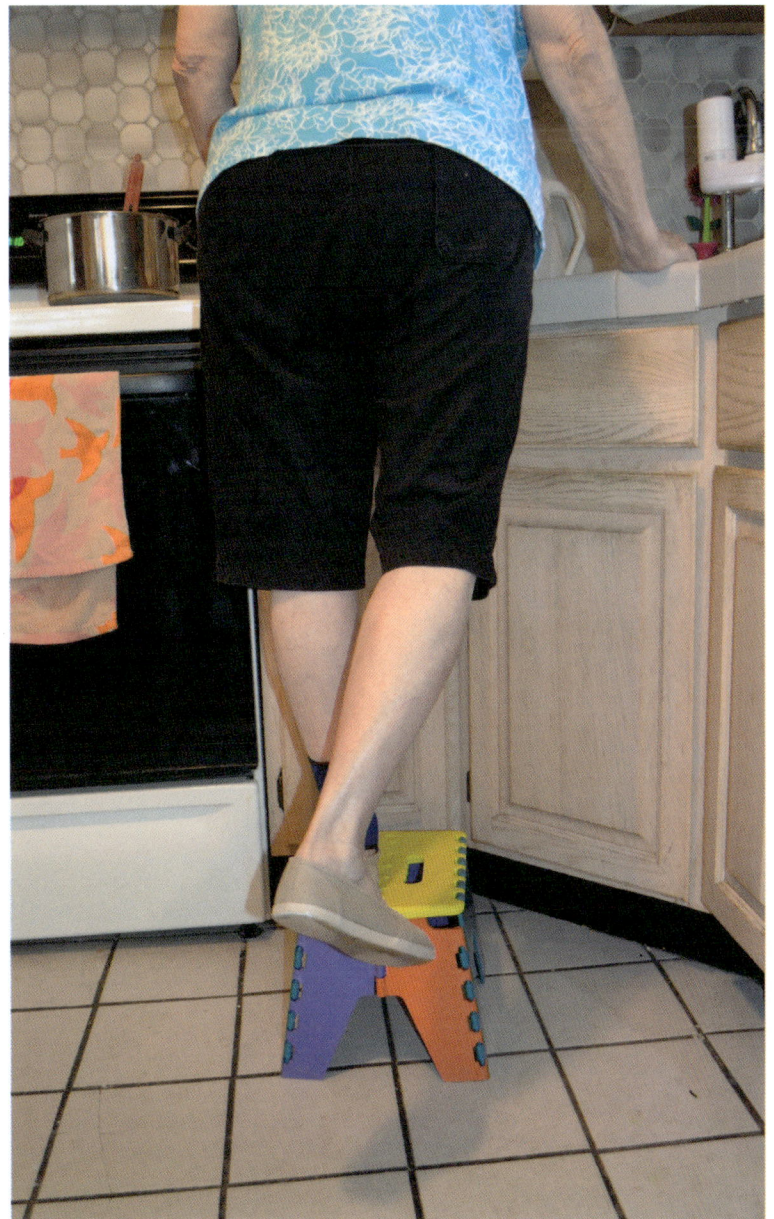

lxix

1.   Explain why this isn't safe.

2.   What would be a better option?

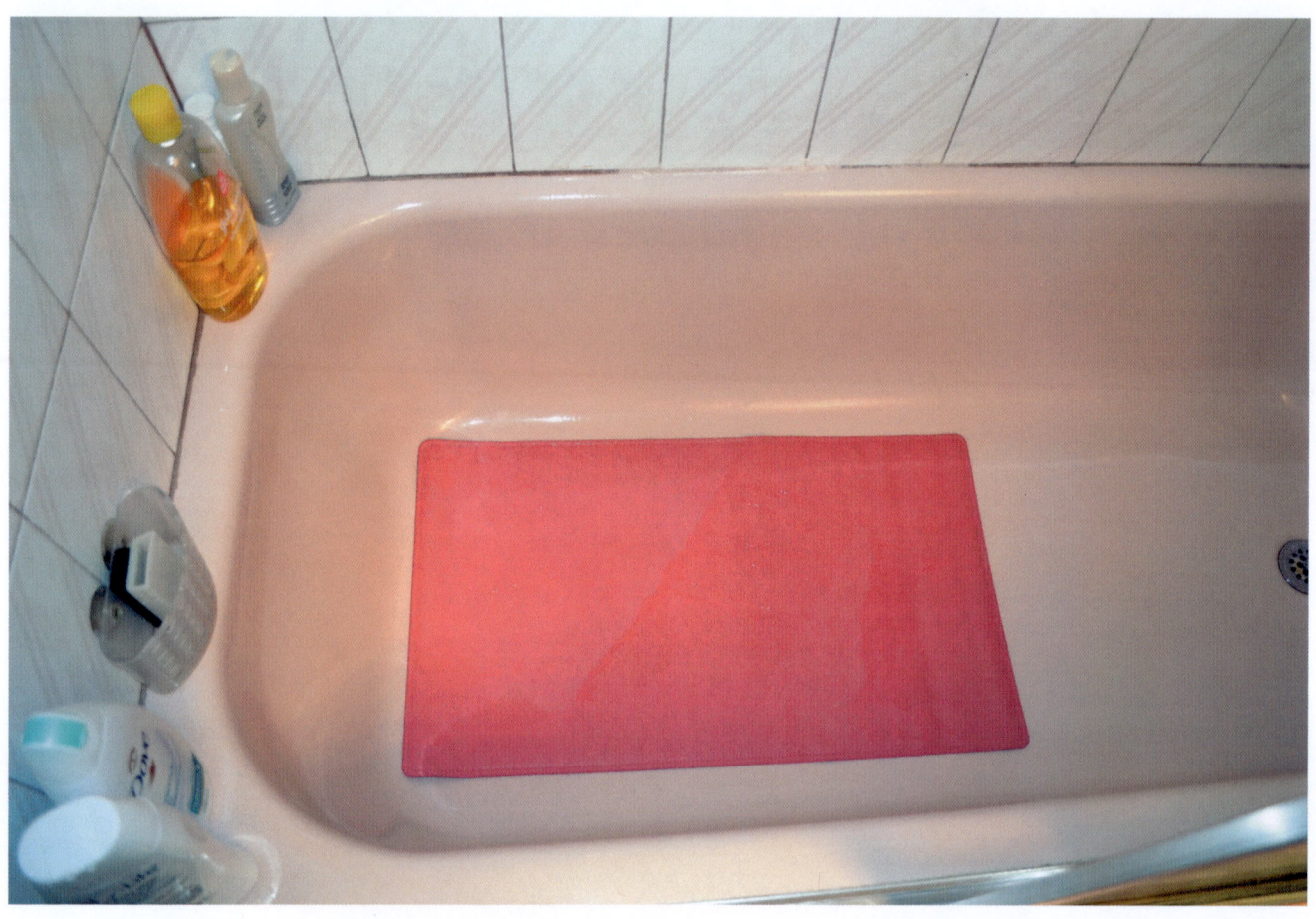

lxx

1. How does this make the tub safer?

2. What other solutions could you use?

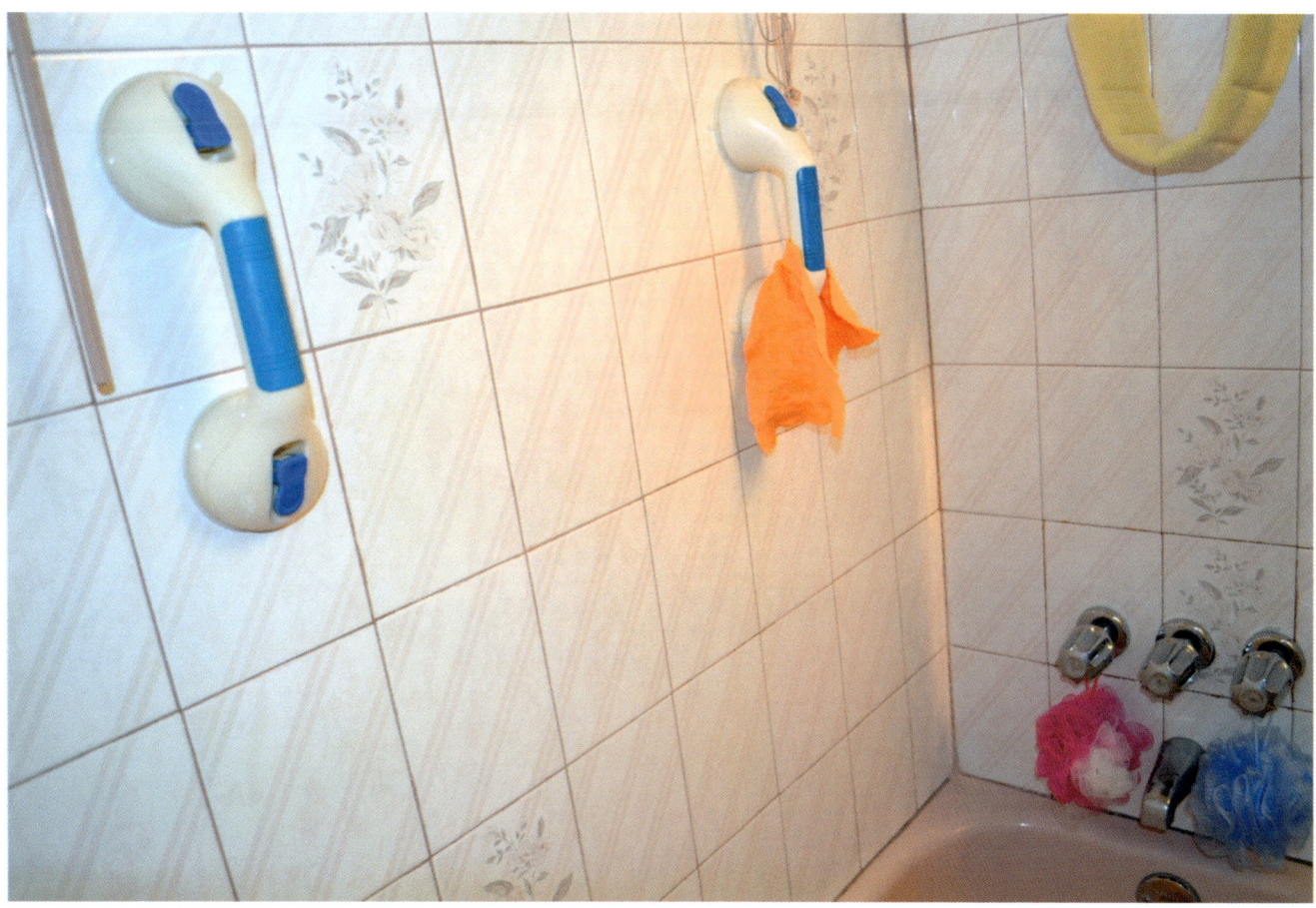

lxxi

1.   What do the hand bars help with in the shower?

2.   What else could you use to prevent falls?

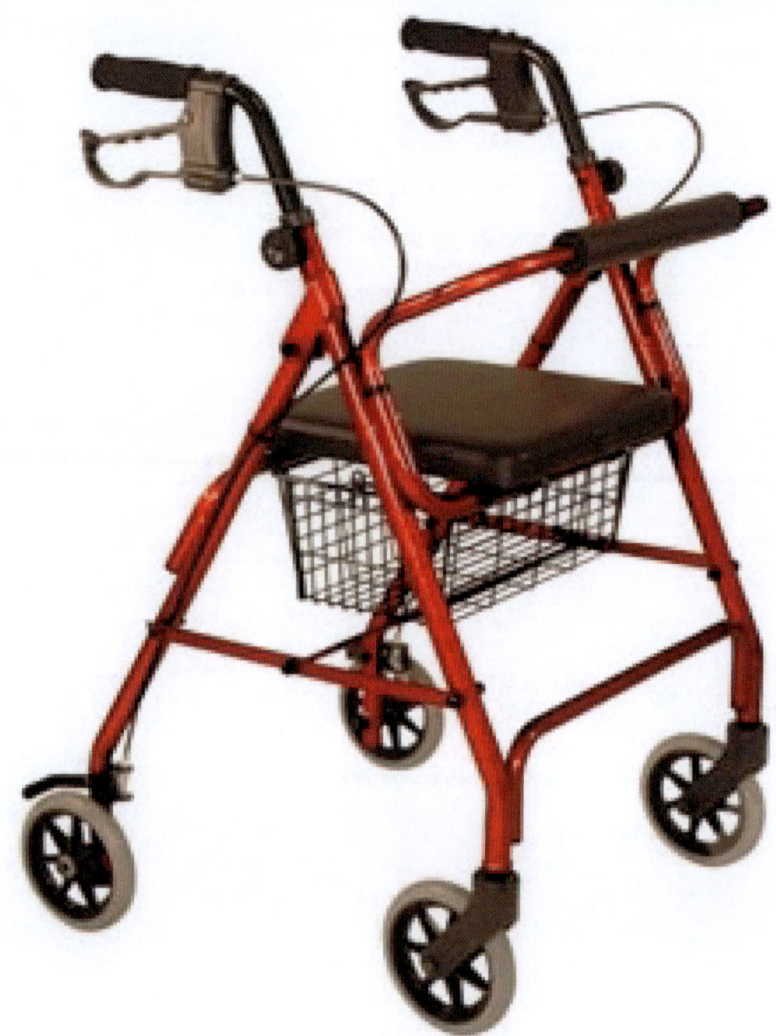

1.   When should somebody use one?

2.   What should you lock before standing up and sitting up?

3.   Explain how to lock the brakes.

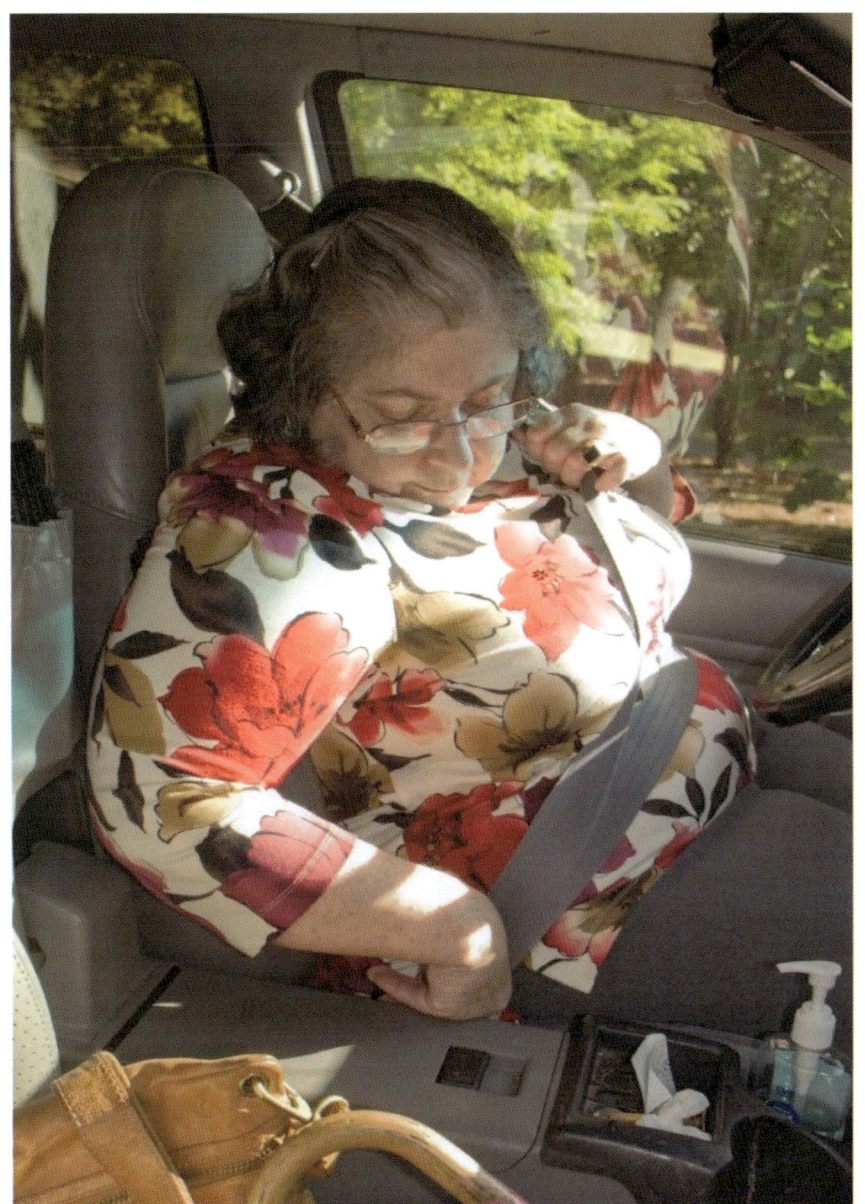

1.   What is she doing?

2.   Why is it safe?

3.   What could happen if she didn't wear her seat belt?

Sequences

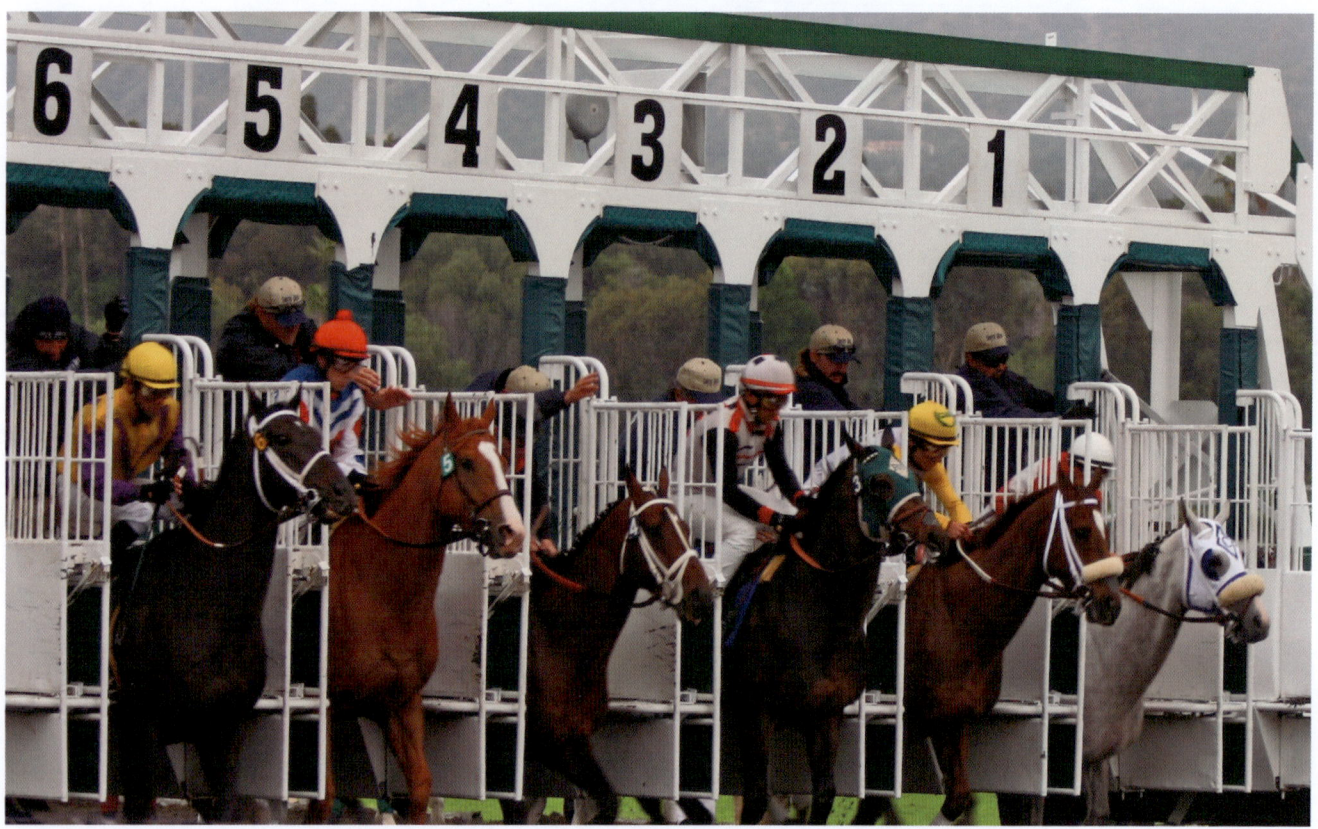

lxxiv

1. What event is this?

2. What does the announcer say?

3. How many horses are there?

4. What is the person called who rides the horse?

5. John went to the race but promised his wife he wouldn't place a bet.

    What type of problem(s) might John have?

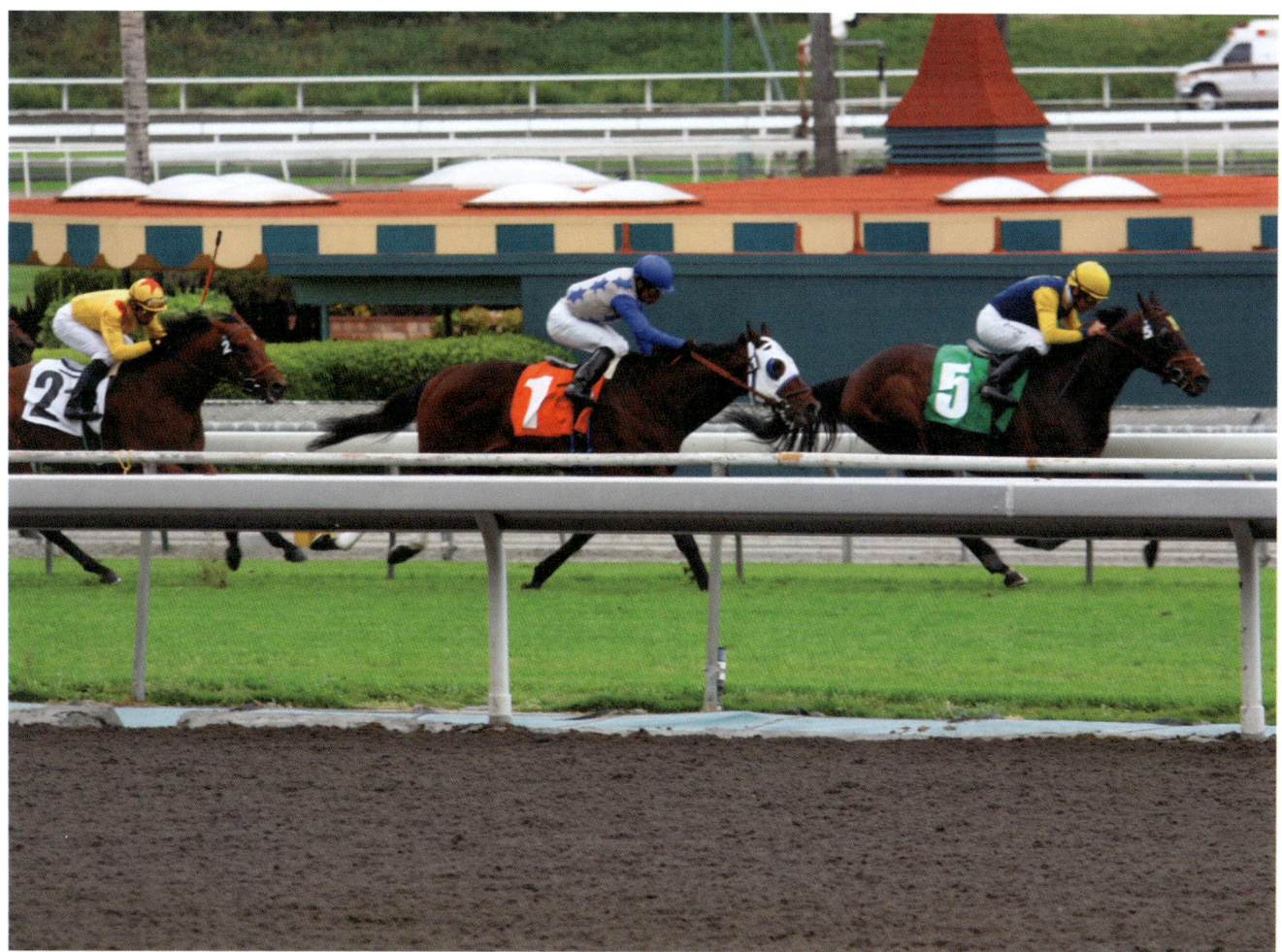

lxxv

1. Describe the photograph.

2. What is it called when a horse runs fast?

3. What is the color and number of the horse in the lead?

4. What colors are the jockey's shirts?

5. There is an ambulance parked in the top right corner of the photo. Why?

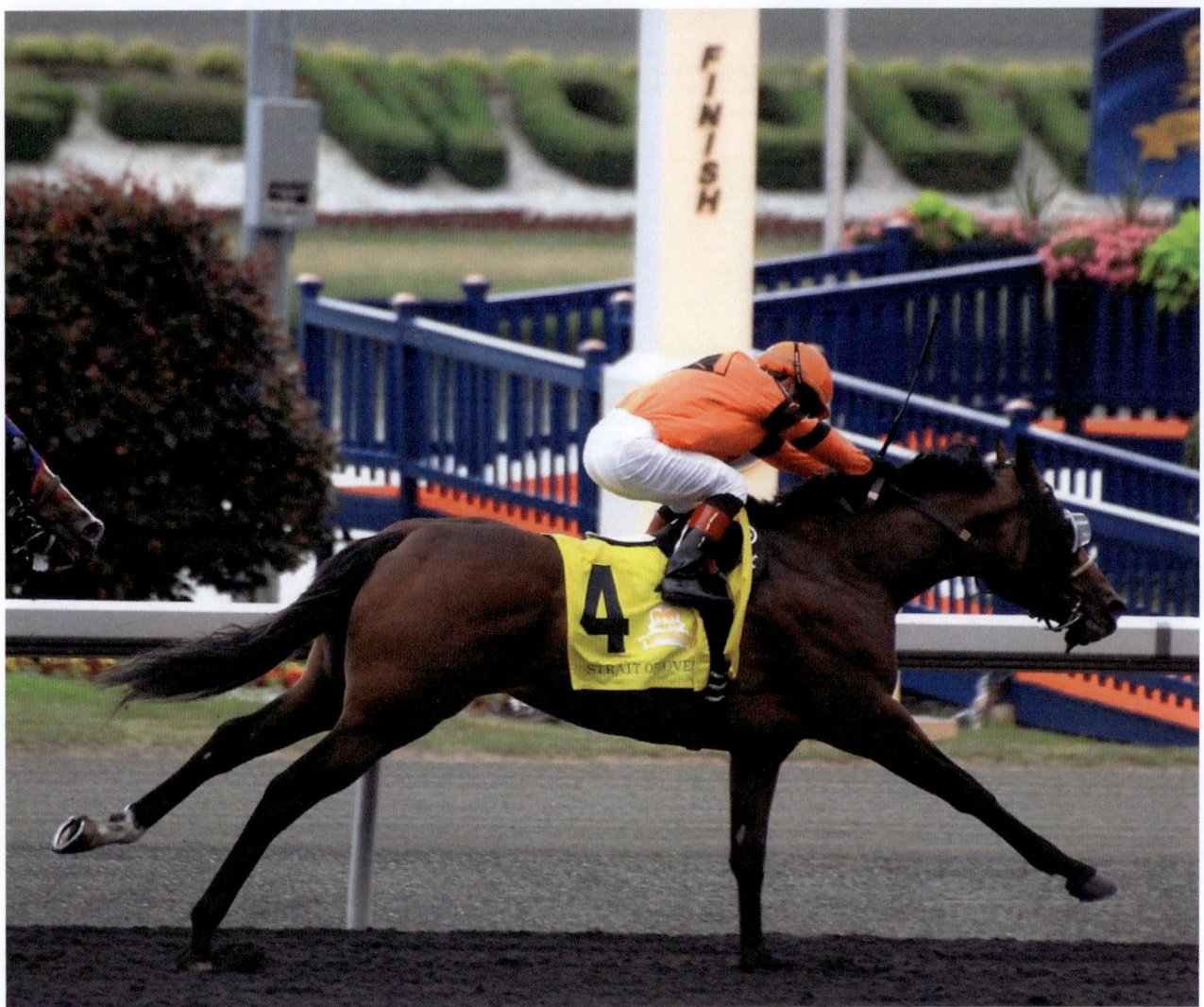

1.   What is this horse doing?

2.   How much do you think the jockey weighs?

3.   Describe the photograph.

4.   Name a famous horse race.

5.   Have you ever been to a horse race

Attack

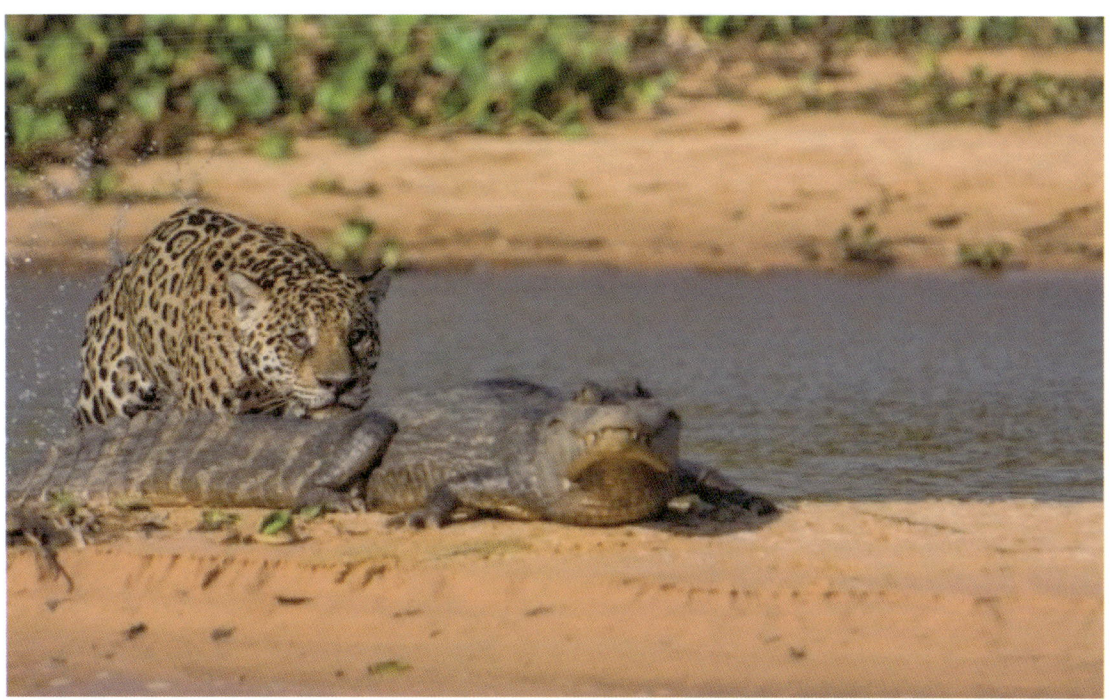

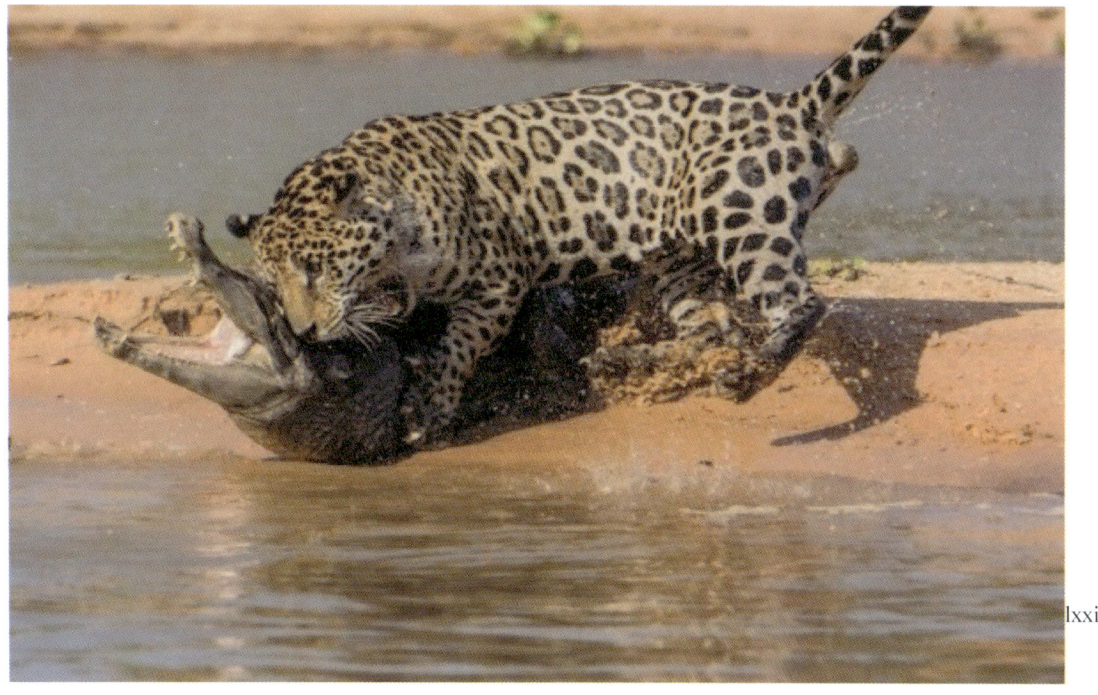

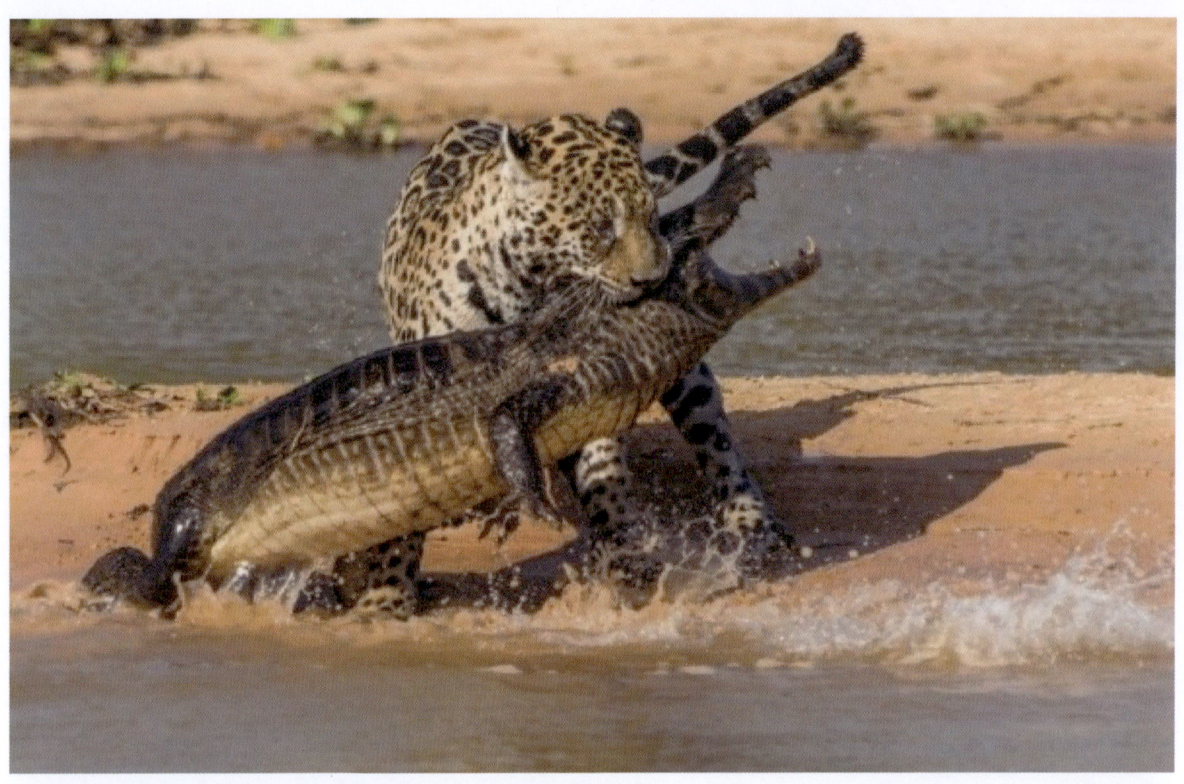

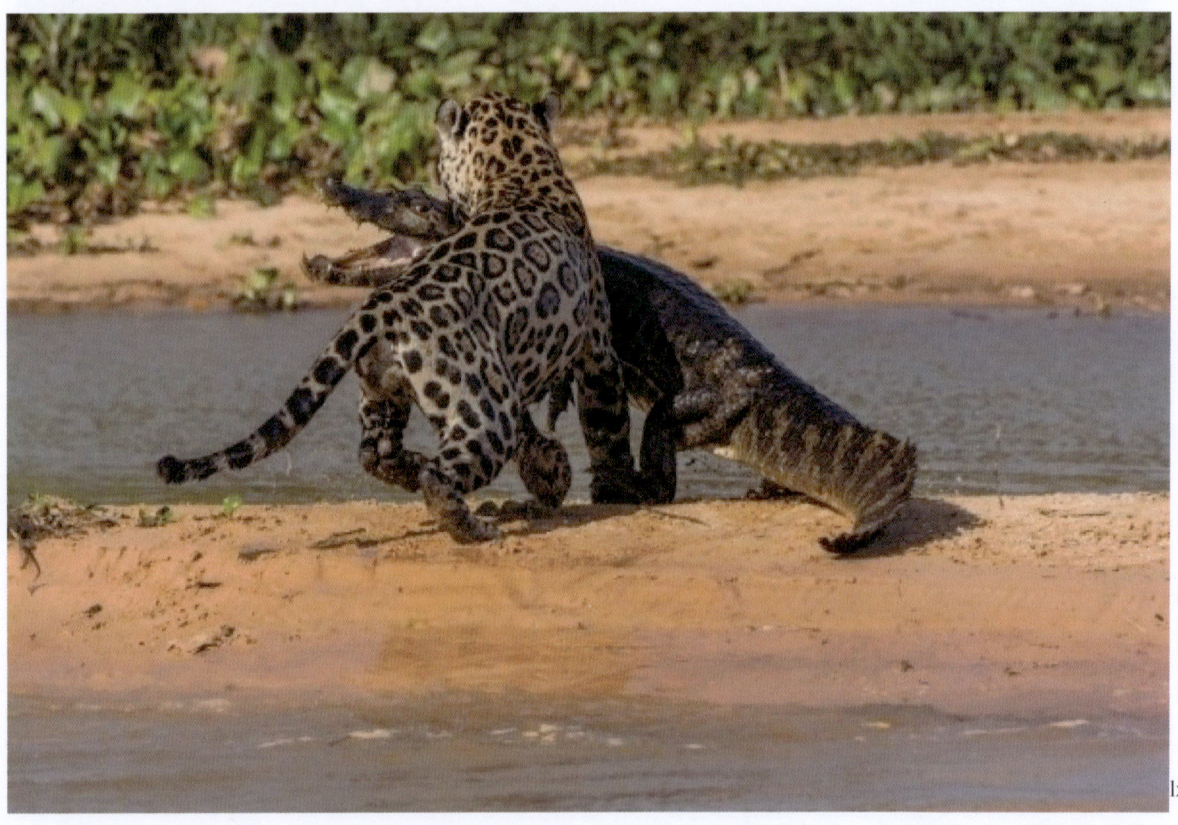

Attack Questions

1. Describe what happened.

2. What animal is hunting?

3. What animal gets attacked?

4. Where is the crocodile?

5. How does the jaguar manage to catch the crocodile?

6. Where does the jaguar bite the crocodile?

7. What will the jaguar do with the crocodile?

8. Was it easy for the jaguar to catch the crocodile? Why? Why not?

9. What continent do you think this took place?

10. Which animal do you think is smarter? Why?

lxxxi

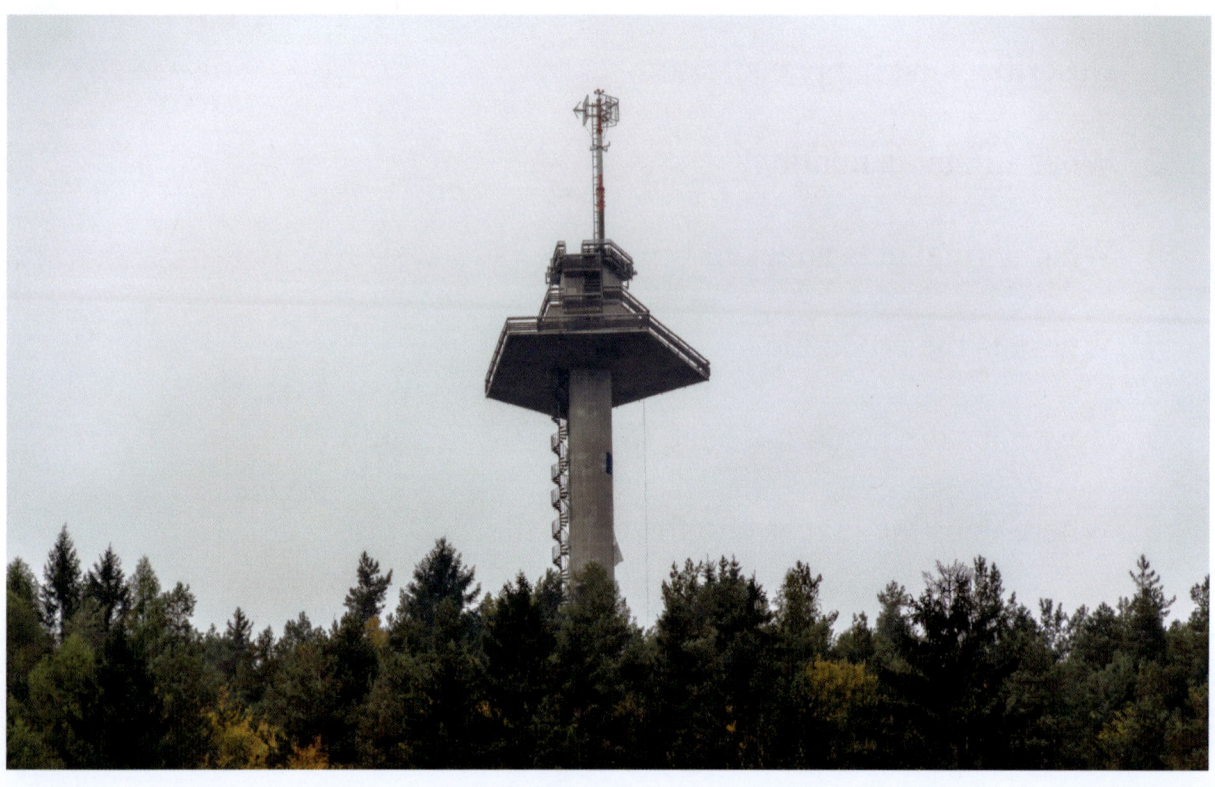

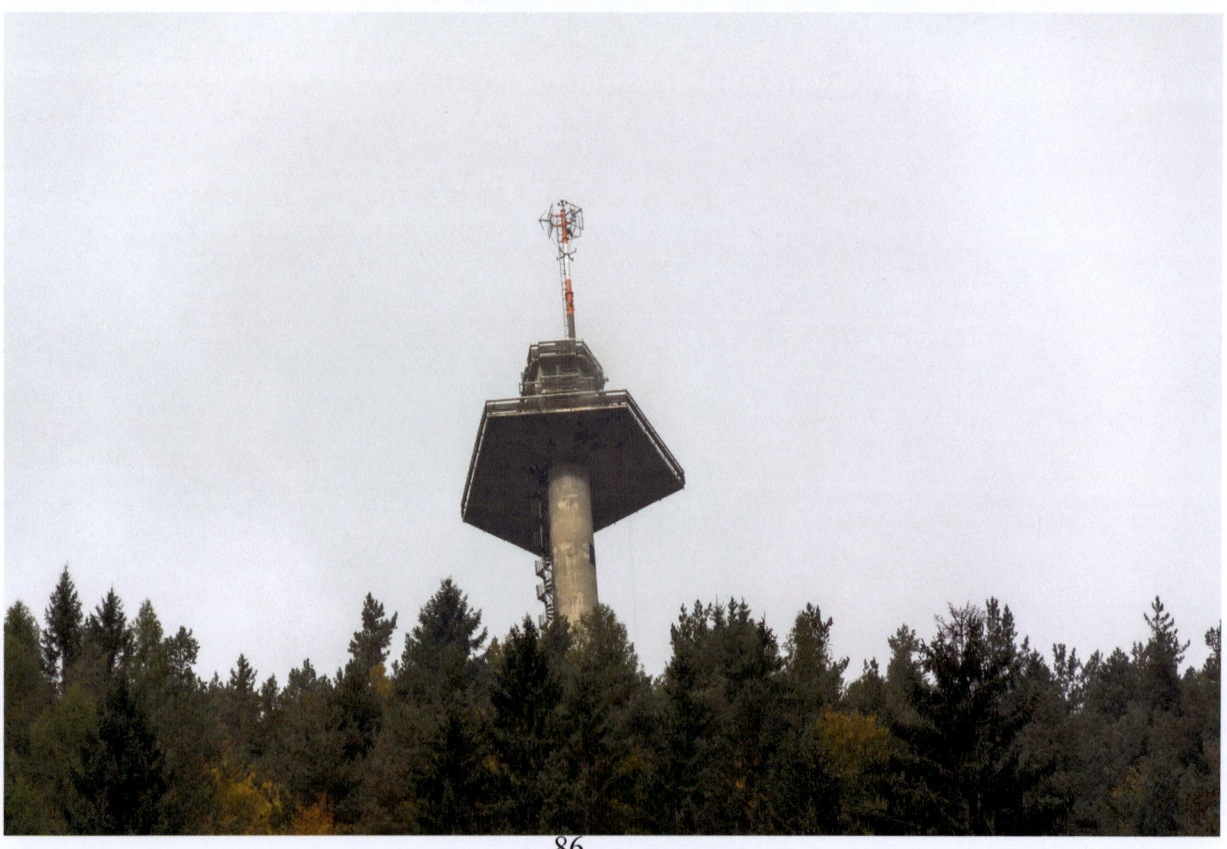

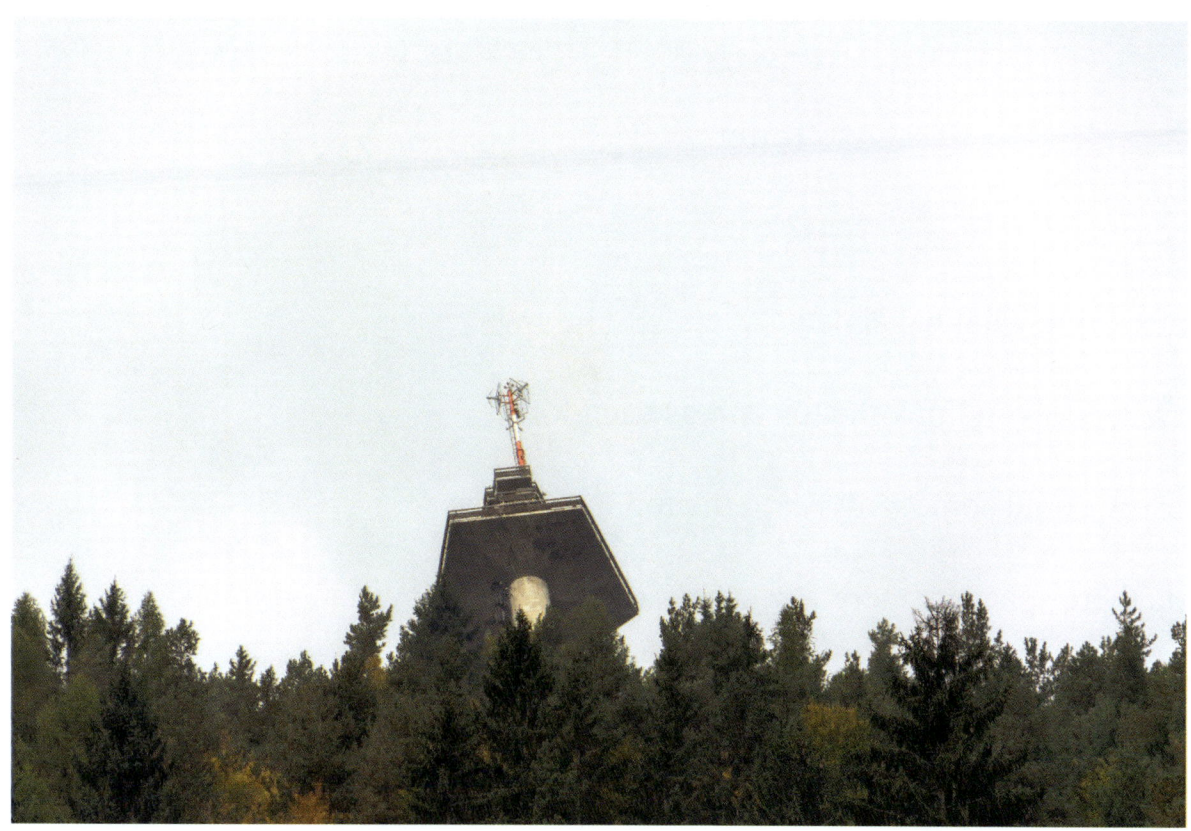

lxxxii

Tower

1. Describe what happened.

2. What do you think the tower was used for?

3. How could somebody get to the top of the tower?

4. Is there space up there for somebody to work? How can you tell?

5. Why do you think it fell down?

6. Describe the tower's surroundings.

7. Show what happened with your hand.

8. If the tower was brought down intentionally, how do you think it was accomplished?

9. If the tower fell as an accident, what do you think could have caused it?

Planting a Flower

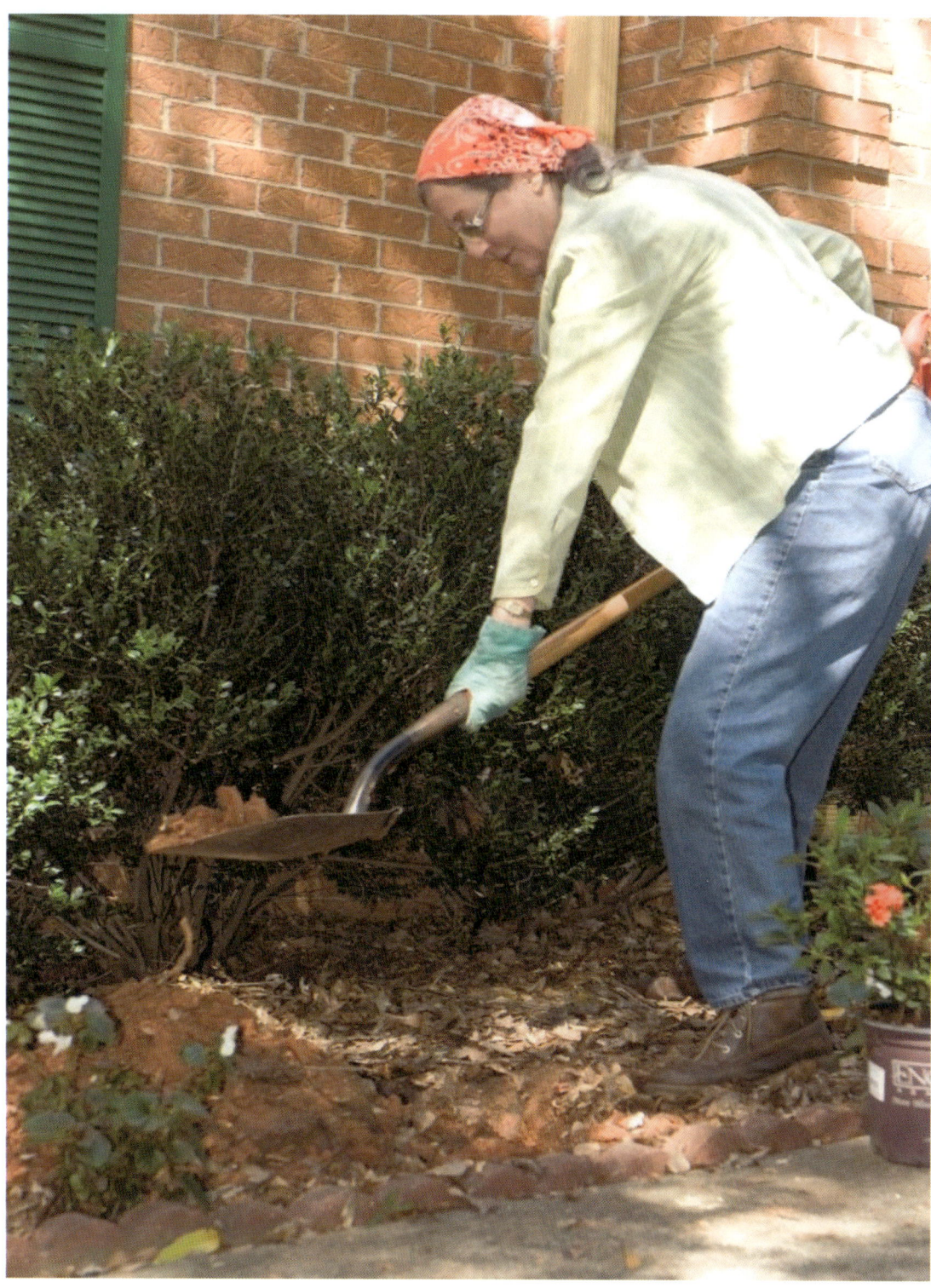

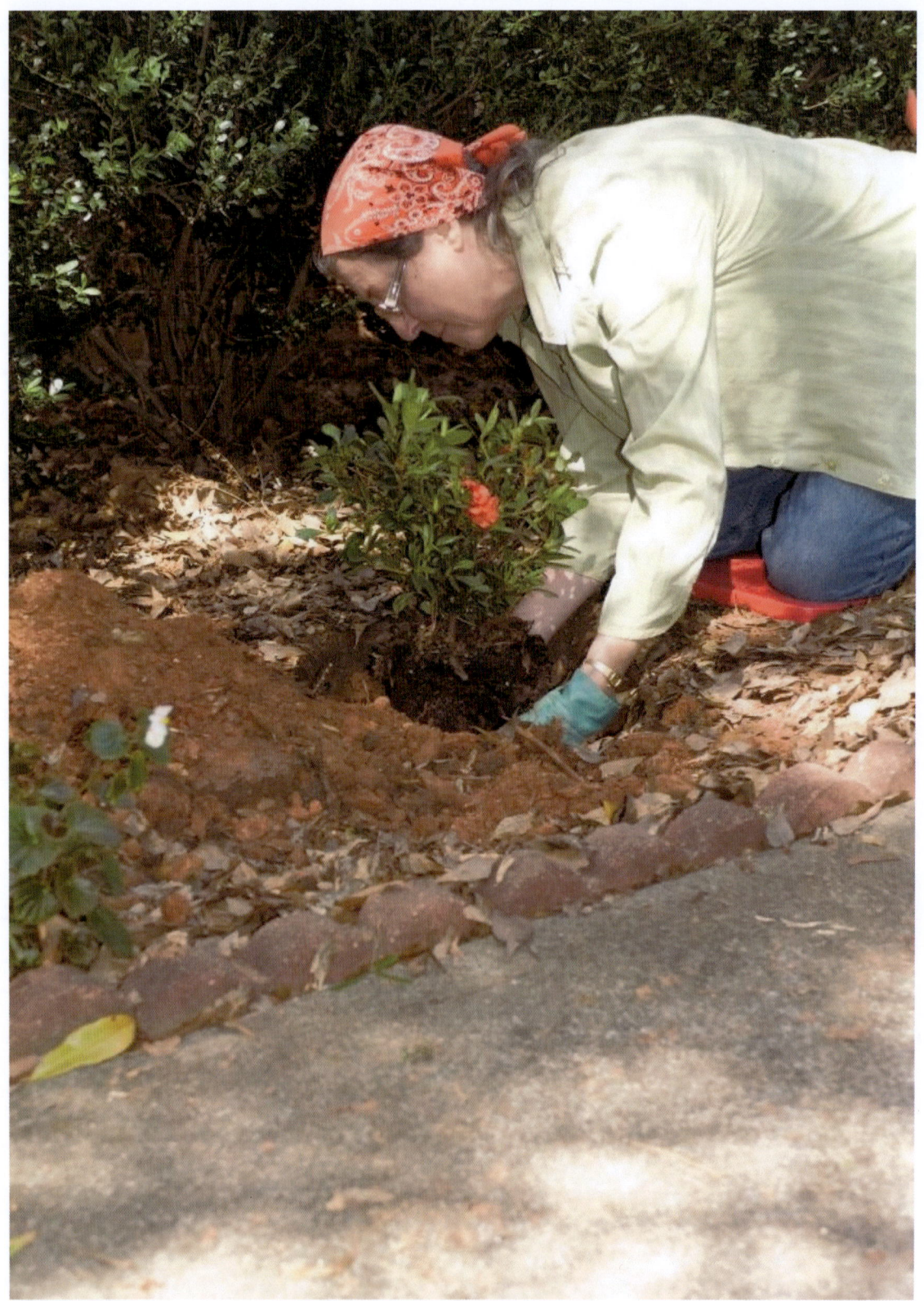

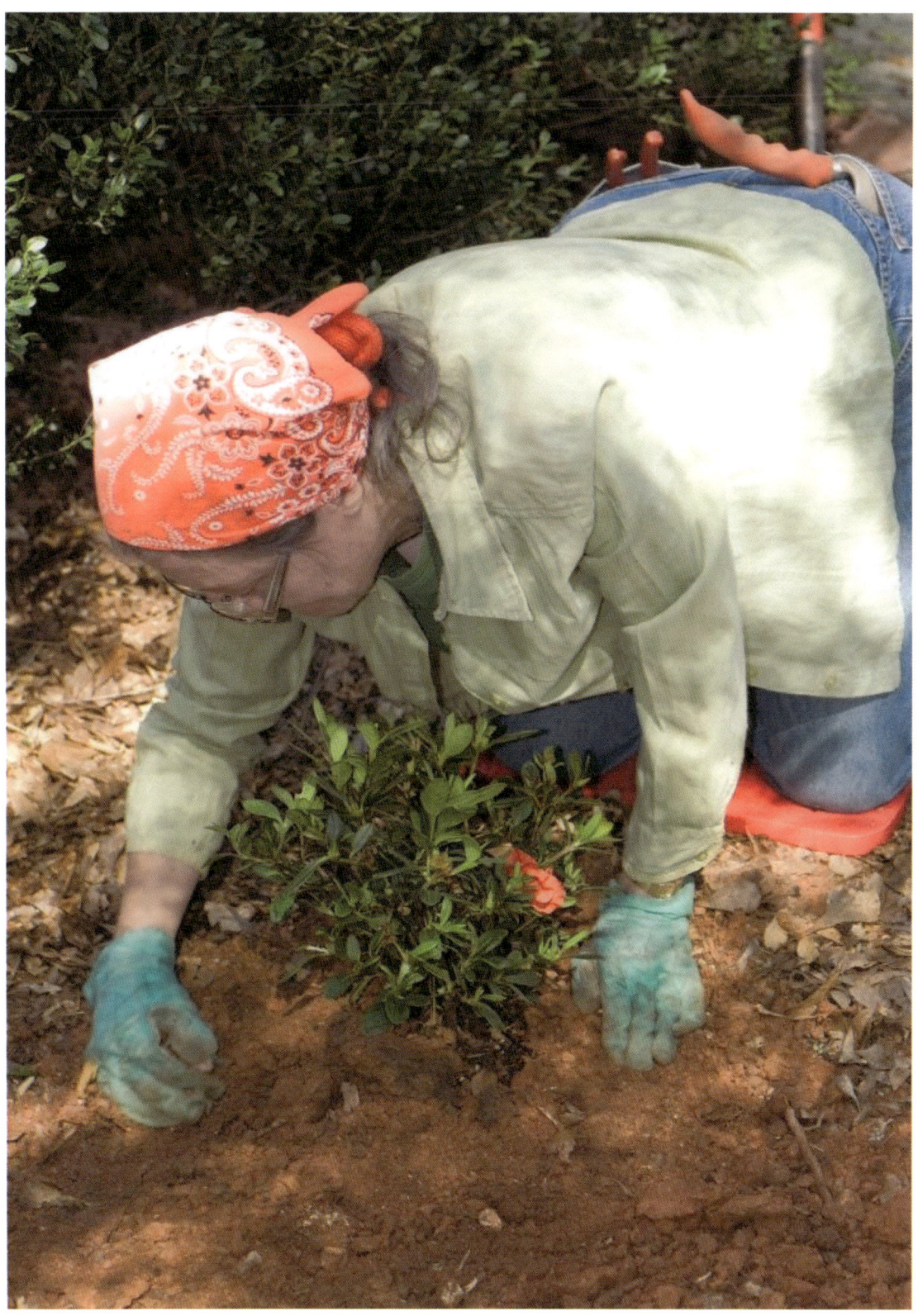

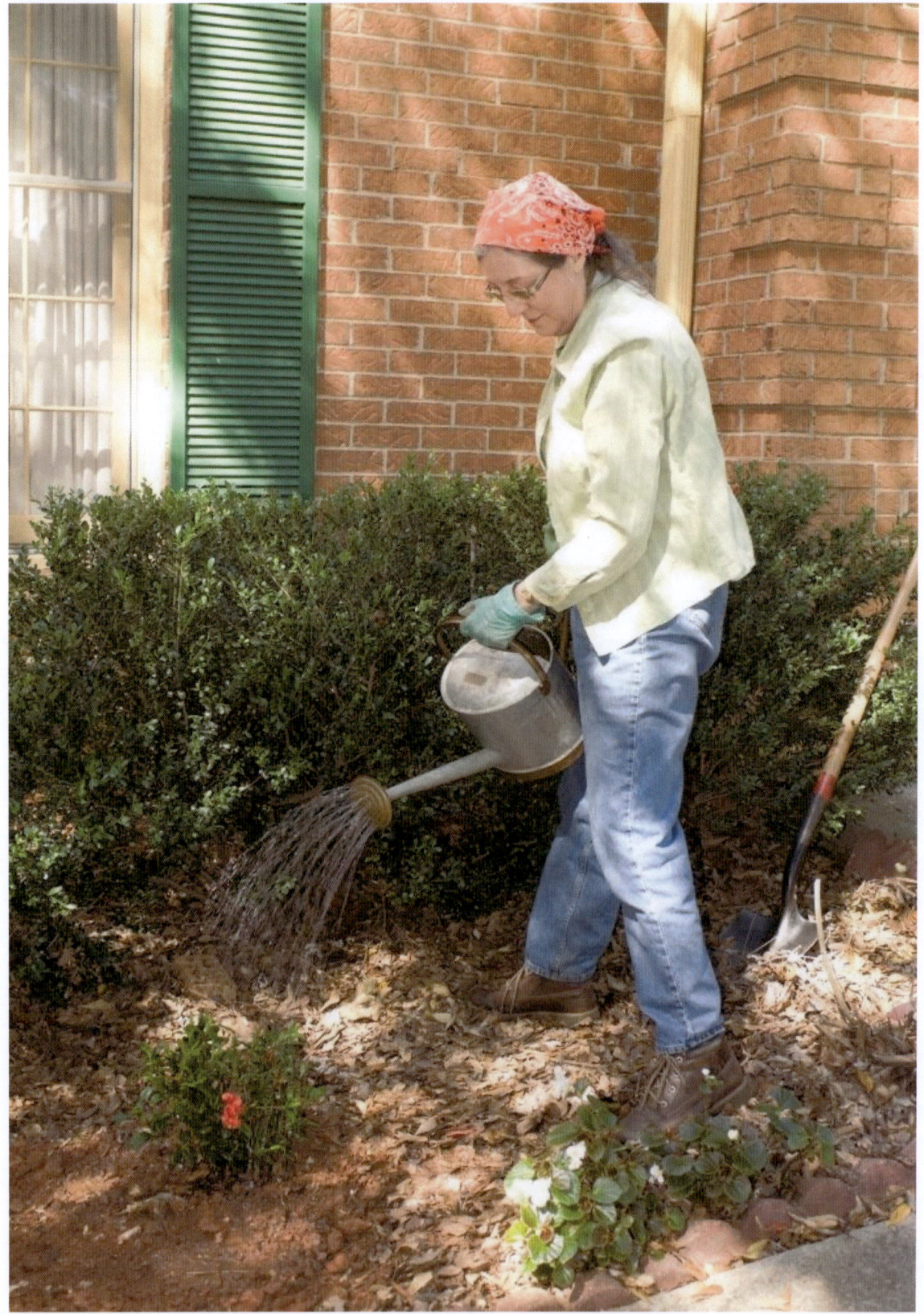

Planting a Flower

1.   Describe the steps to complete the task.

2.   What does a plant need to grow?

3.   Where did she plant the flower?

4.   What is the difference between annuals and perennials?

5.   What tools did she use to plant the flower?

6.   What type of plant did she have?

7.   What time of year is it?

8.   Describe what she is wearing.

9.   What does it mean to have a green thumb?

10.   What have you grown in your yard?

Crossing the Street

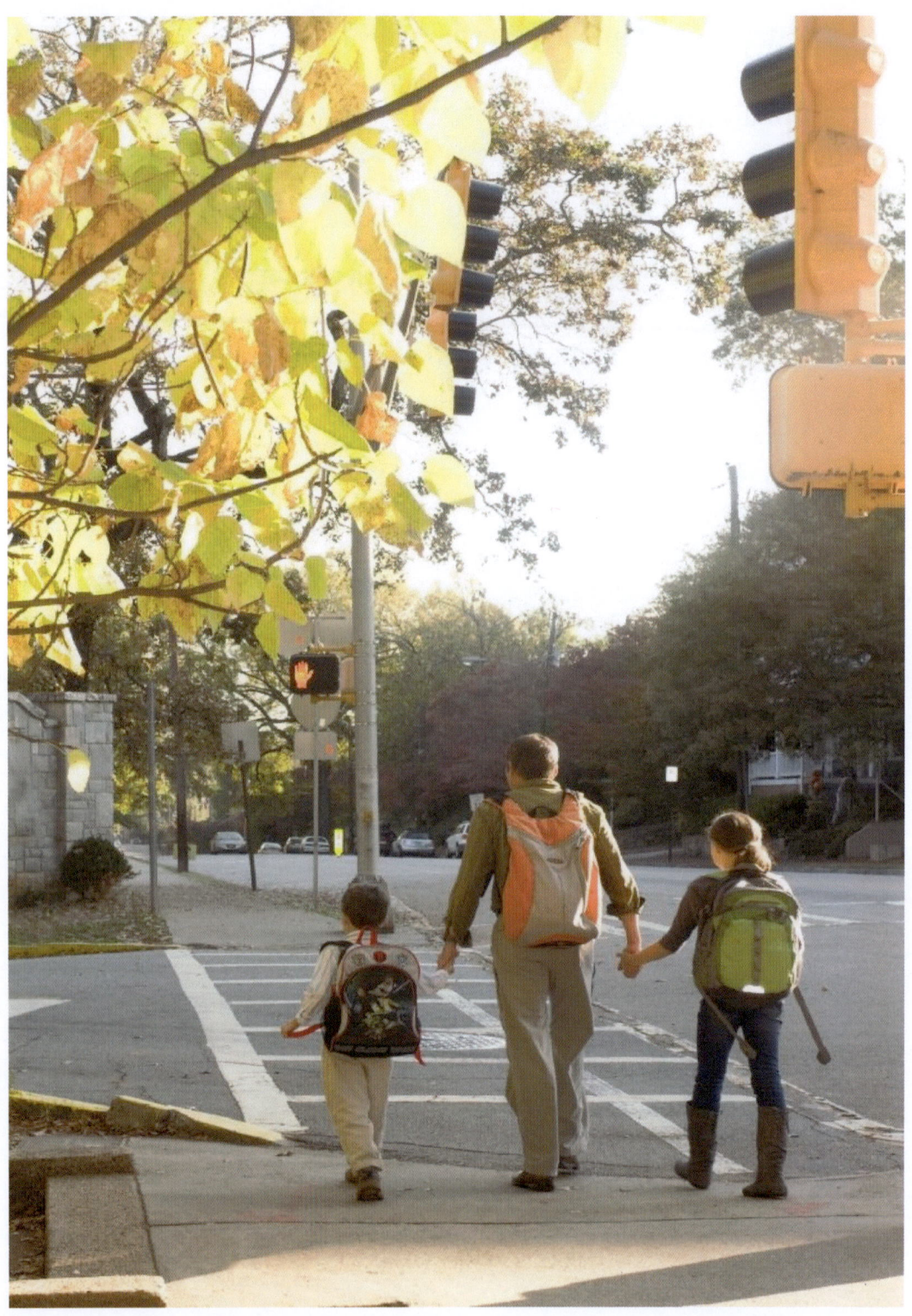

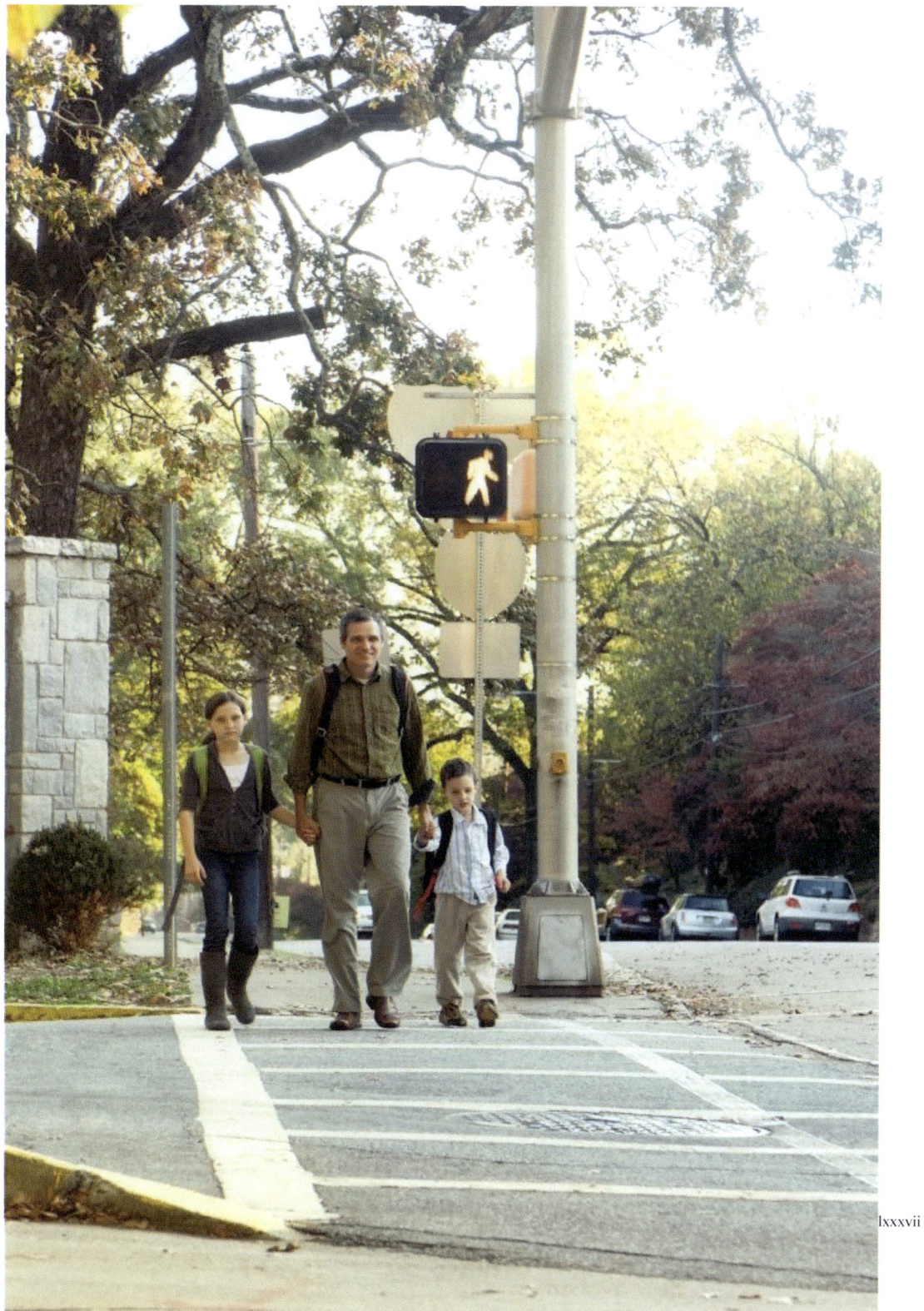

lxxxvii

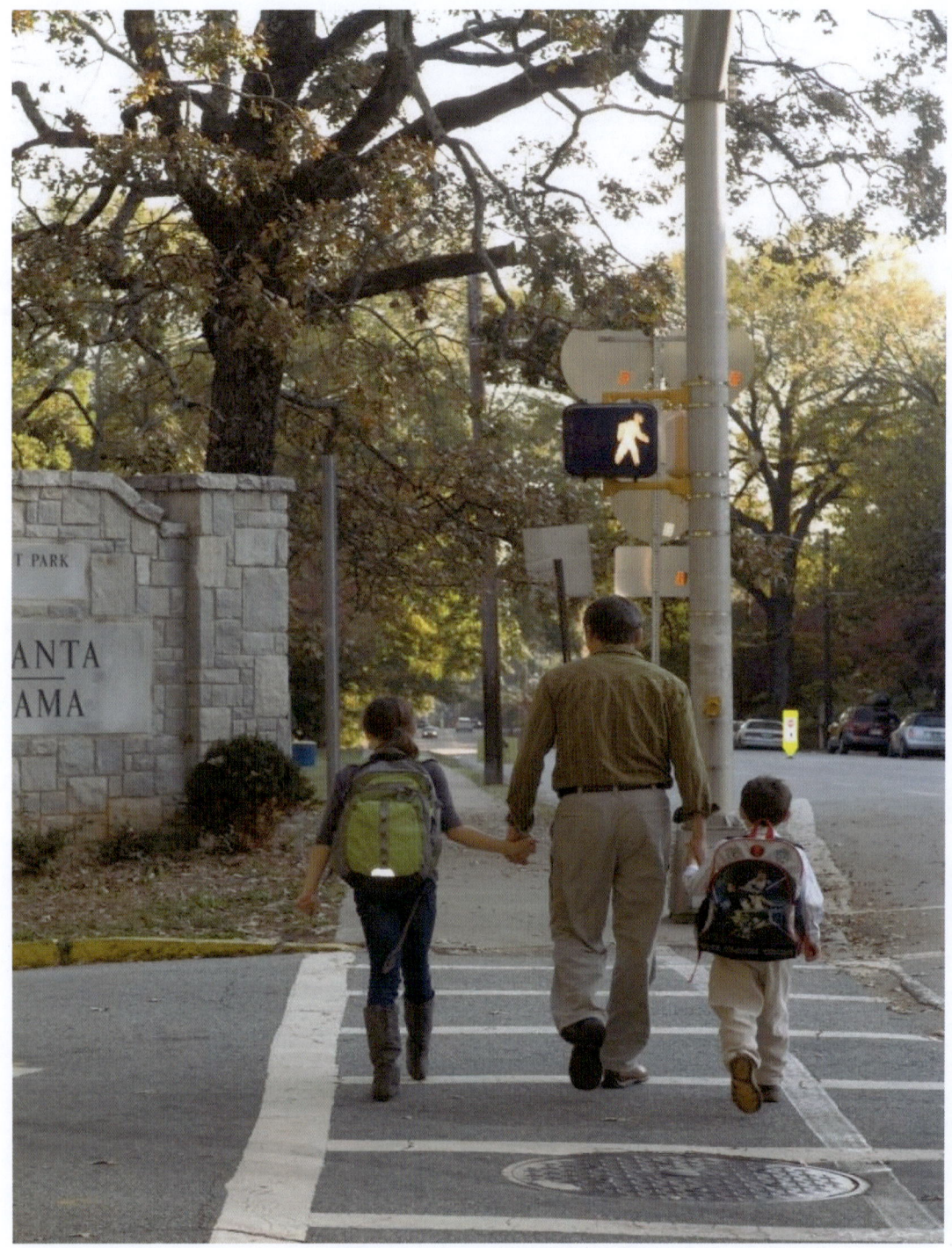

1. Describe the action in the sequence of photos.

2. What did they do safely?

3. Can you find two things that are different in the last photo?

Cleaning a Fish

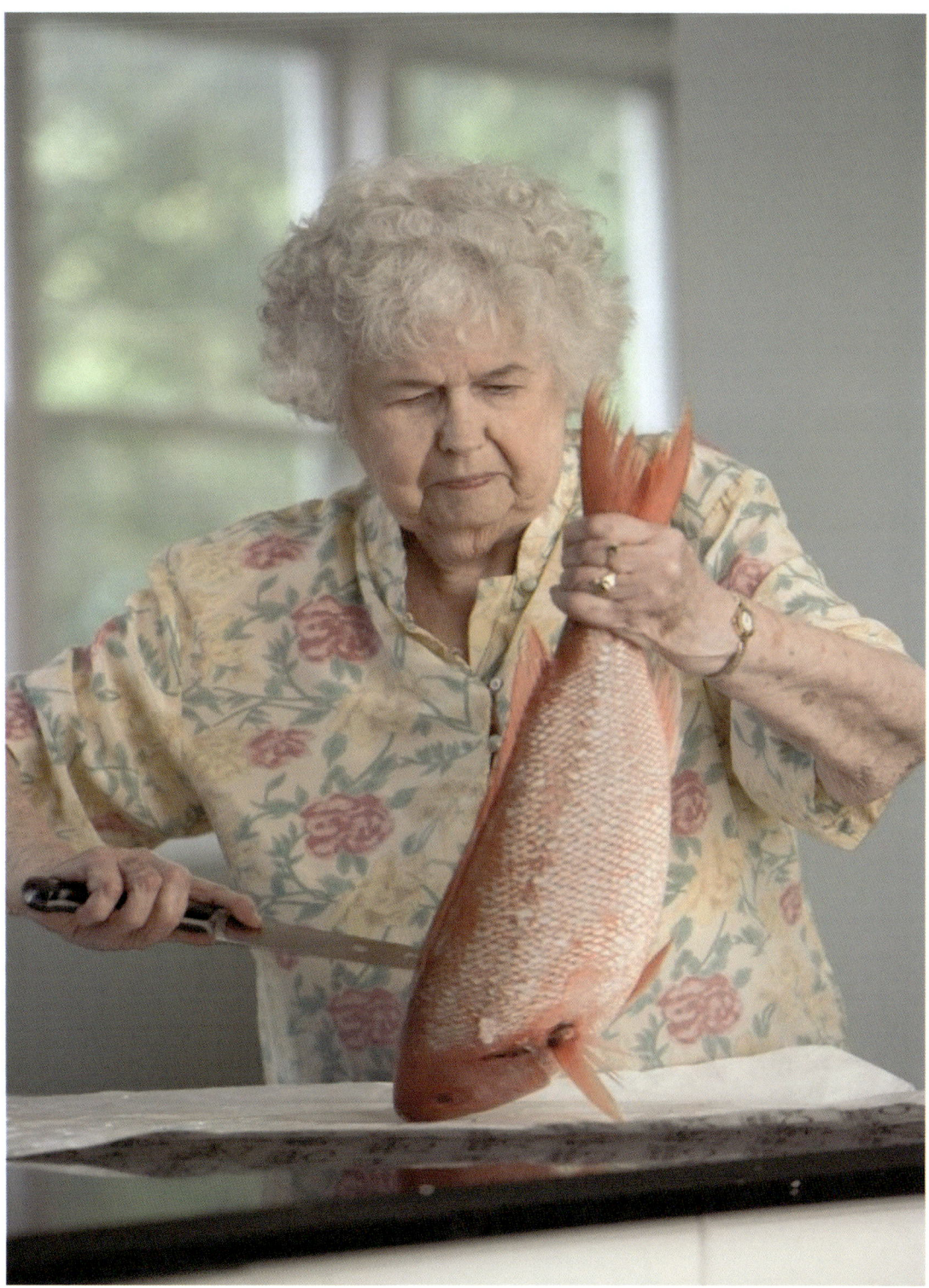

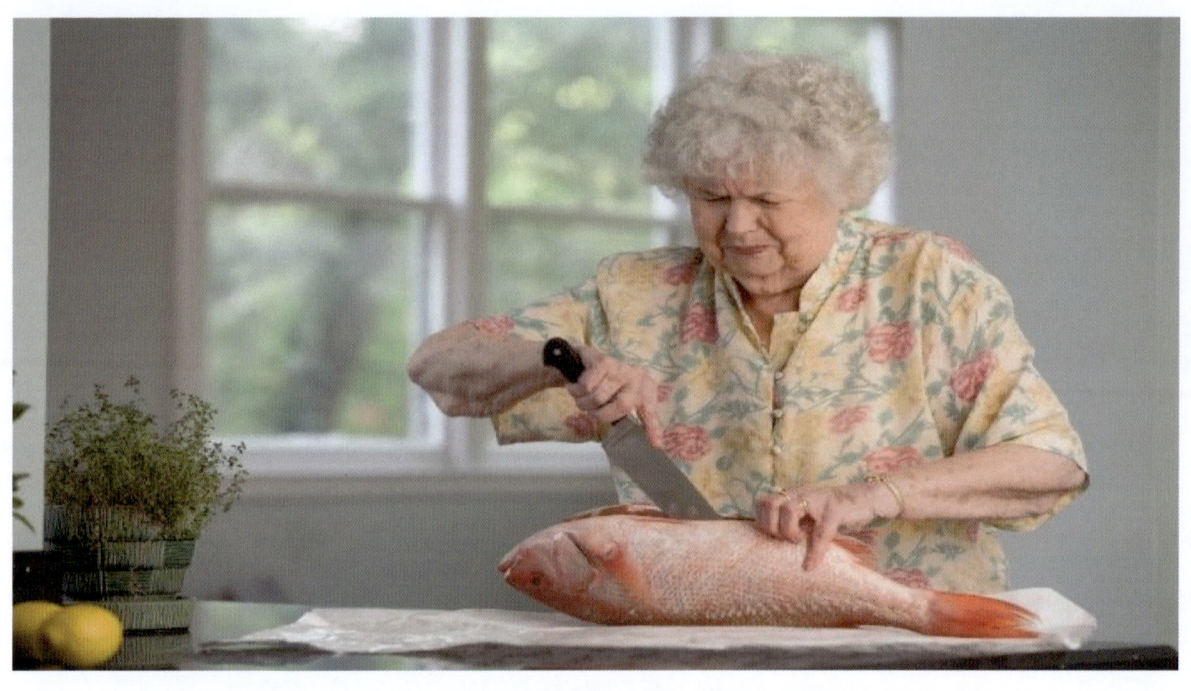

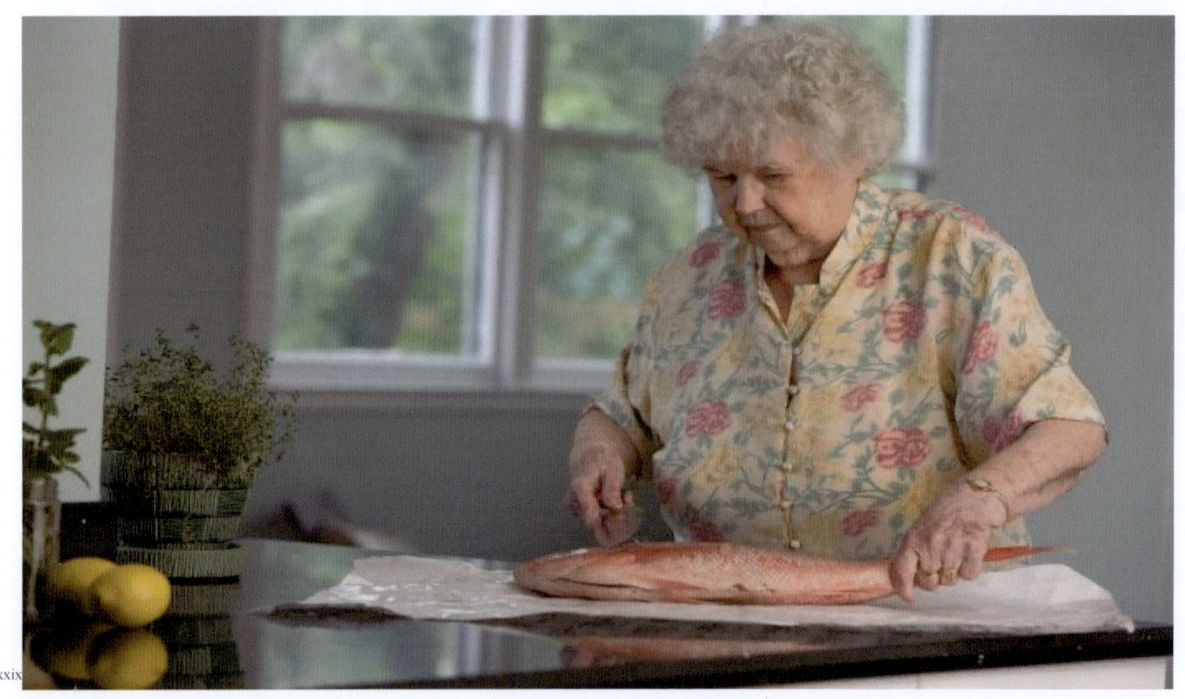

Cleaning a Fish

1.   Describe the lady who cleaned the fish?

2.   Do you think she caught the fish? Why? Why Not?

3.   If she didn't catch the fish, who did?

4.   What are the steps required in cleaning a fish?

5.   Have you ever cleaned a fish?

6.   Describe what this lady is doing.

7.   Describe her expression in the second photograph.

8.   What items are on her counter top?

9.   What is your favorite kind of seafood?

10.   Show a gesture pretending to fish.

Describing Items

Cakes

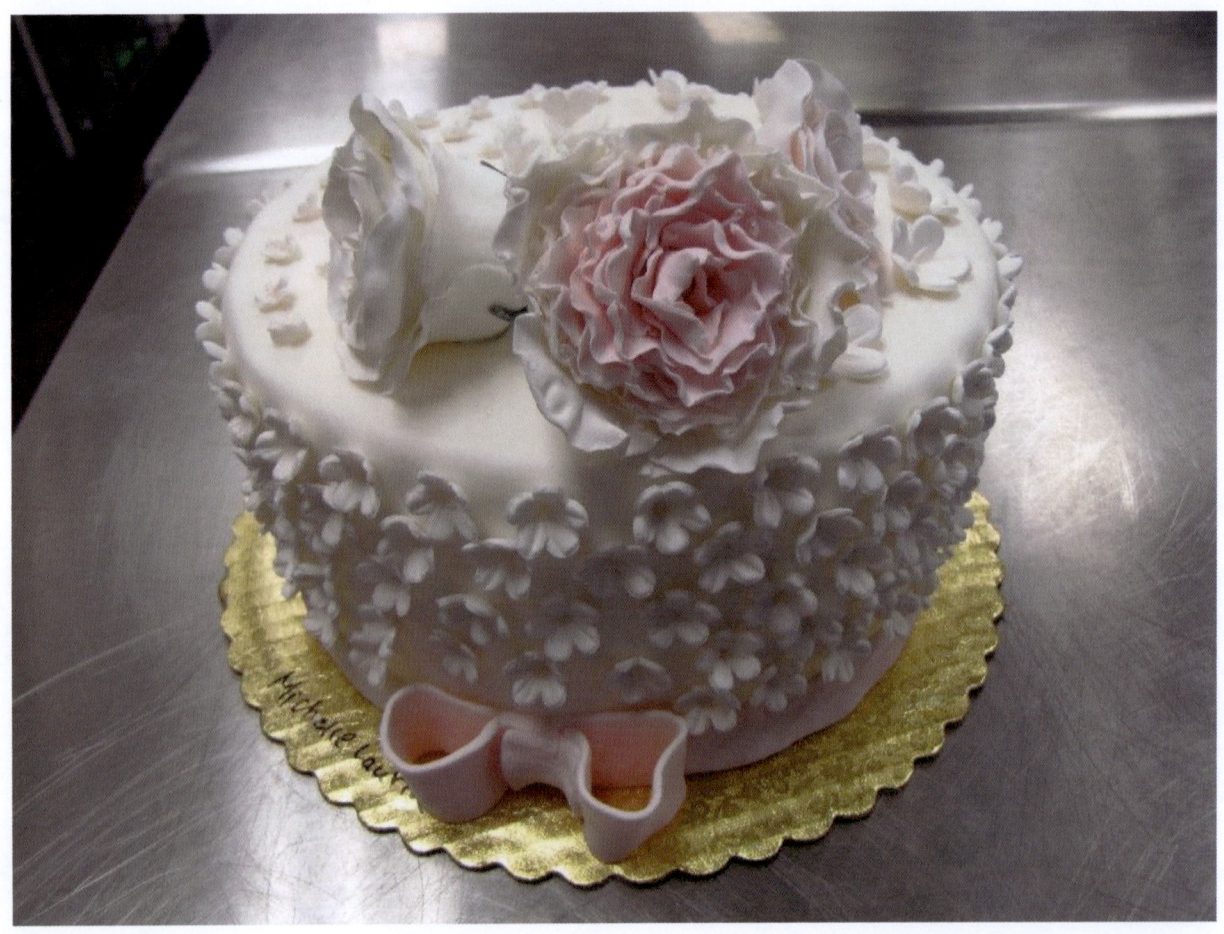

Describe each cake and then answer the questions for every cake.

1. What flavor do you think it is?

2. For what occasion could this cake be for?

3. How long do you think it took to make this cake?

4. How much do you think each cake costs?

5. Which cake is your favorite?

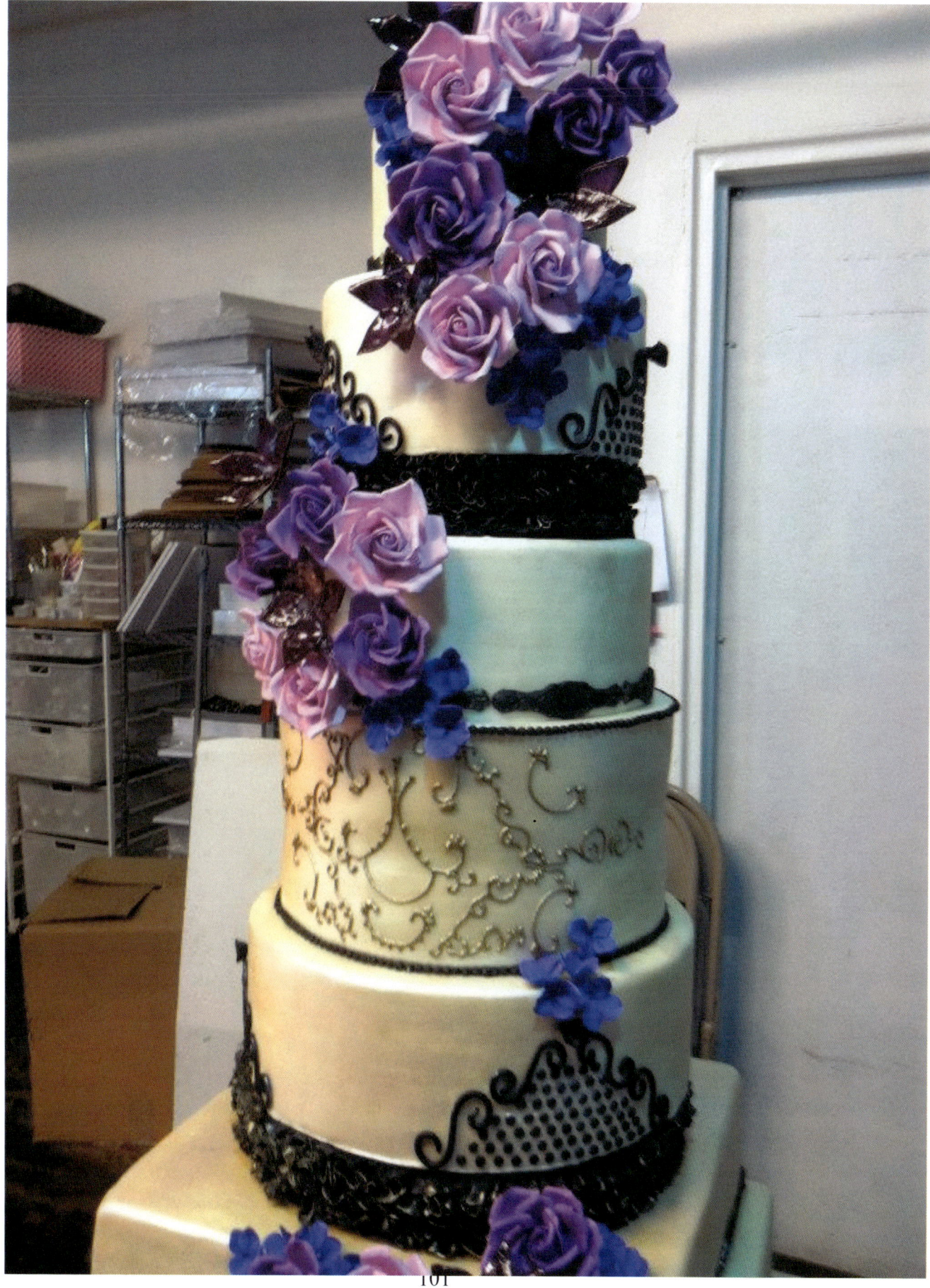

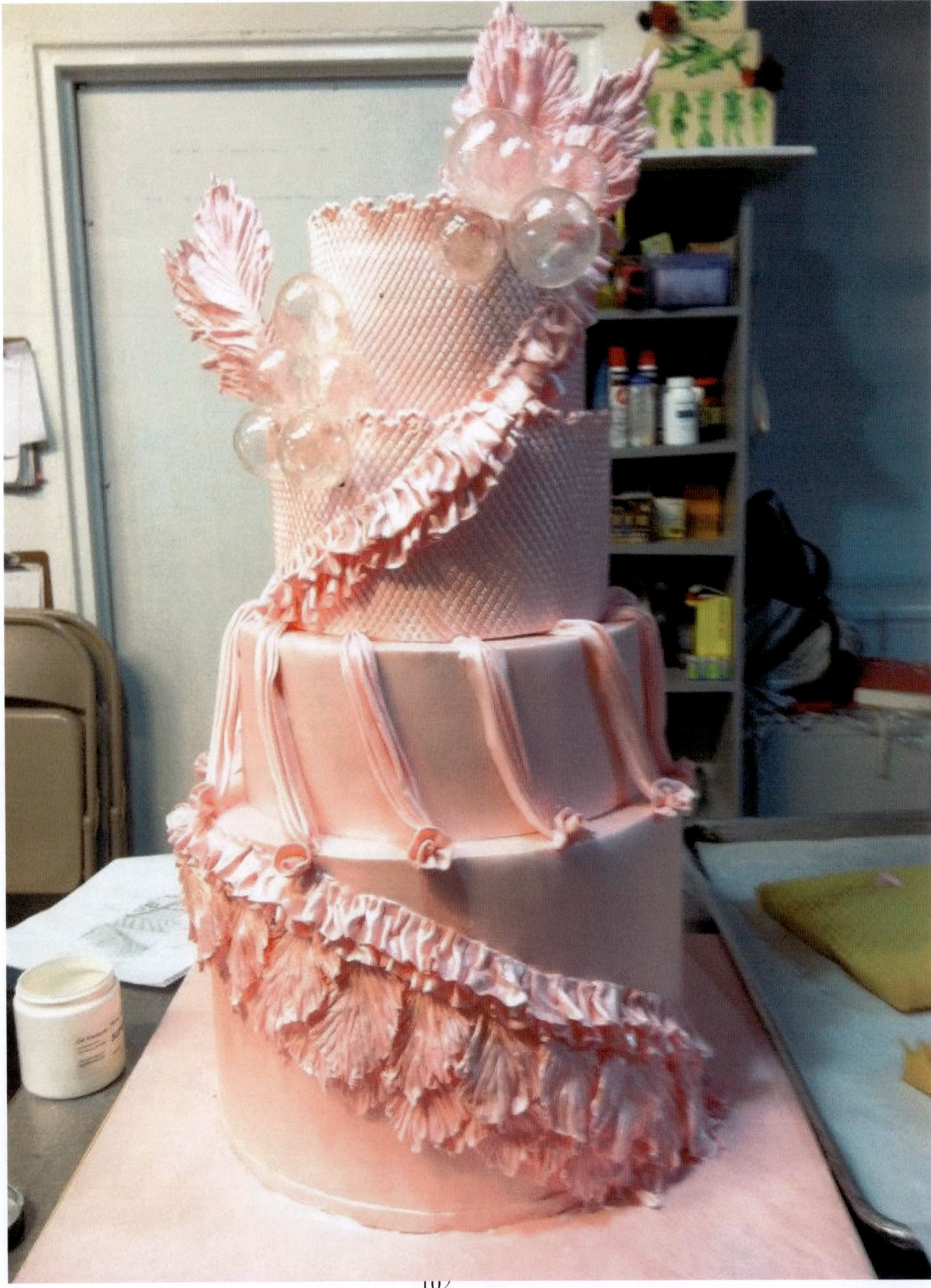

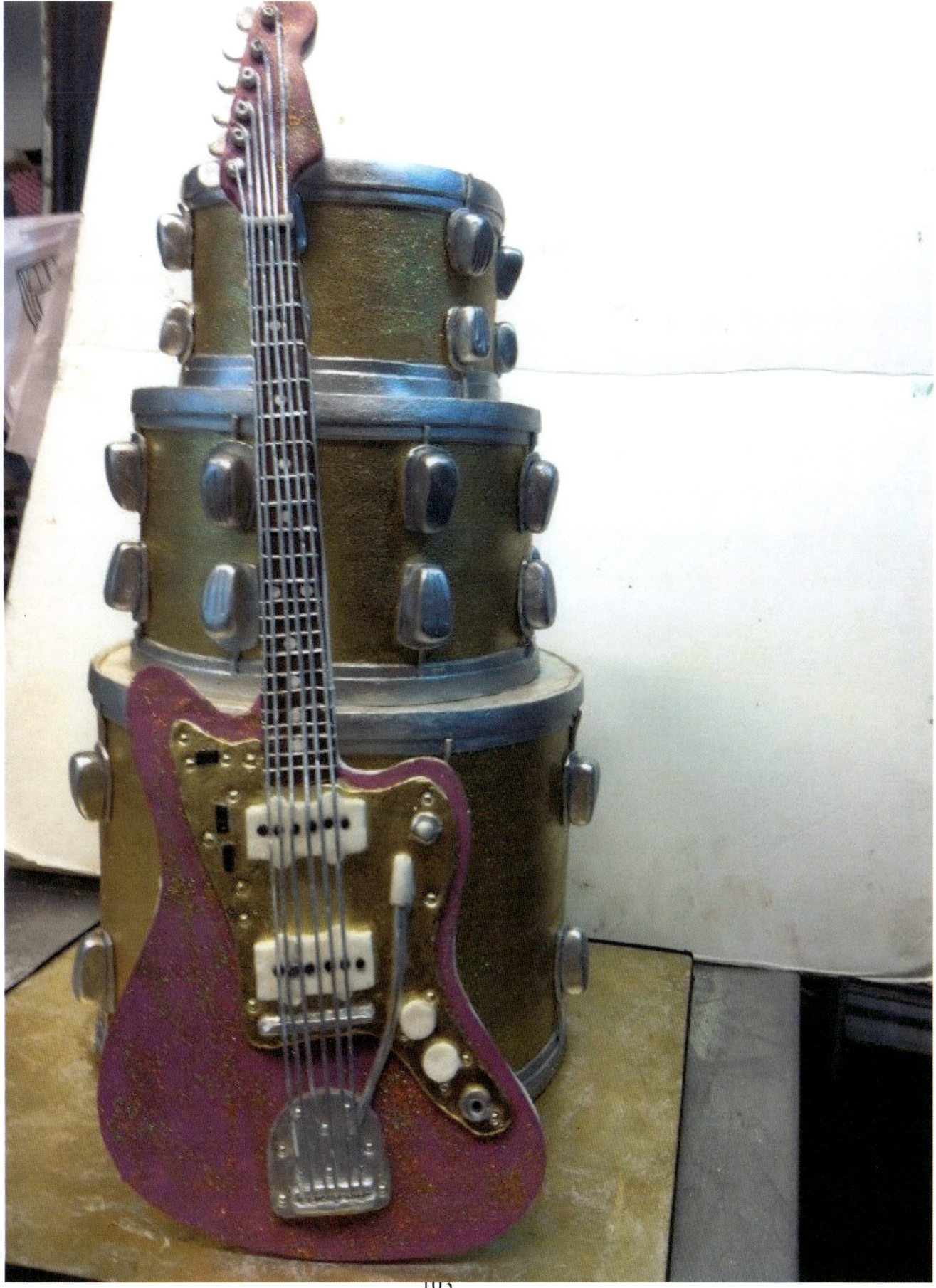

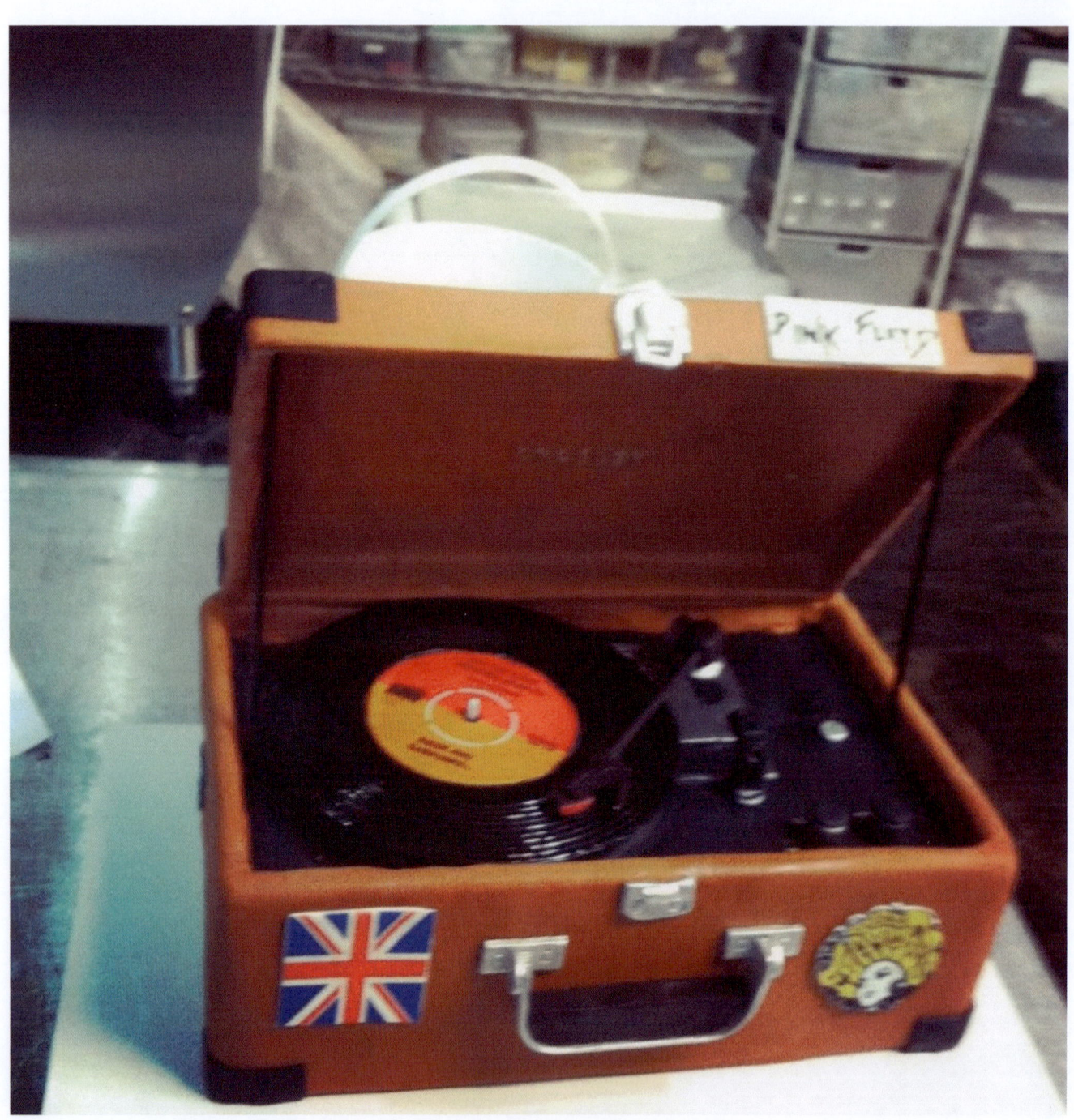

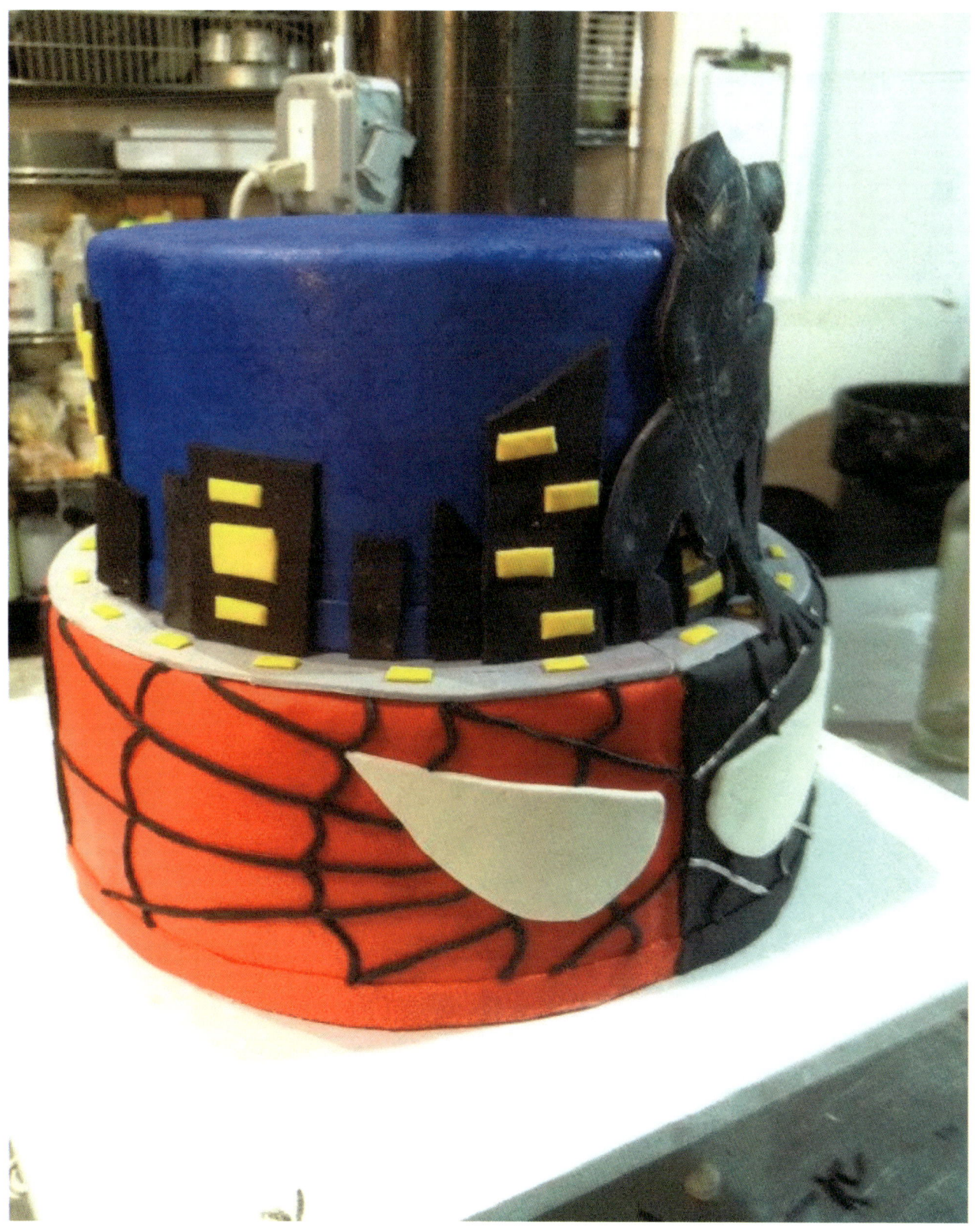

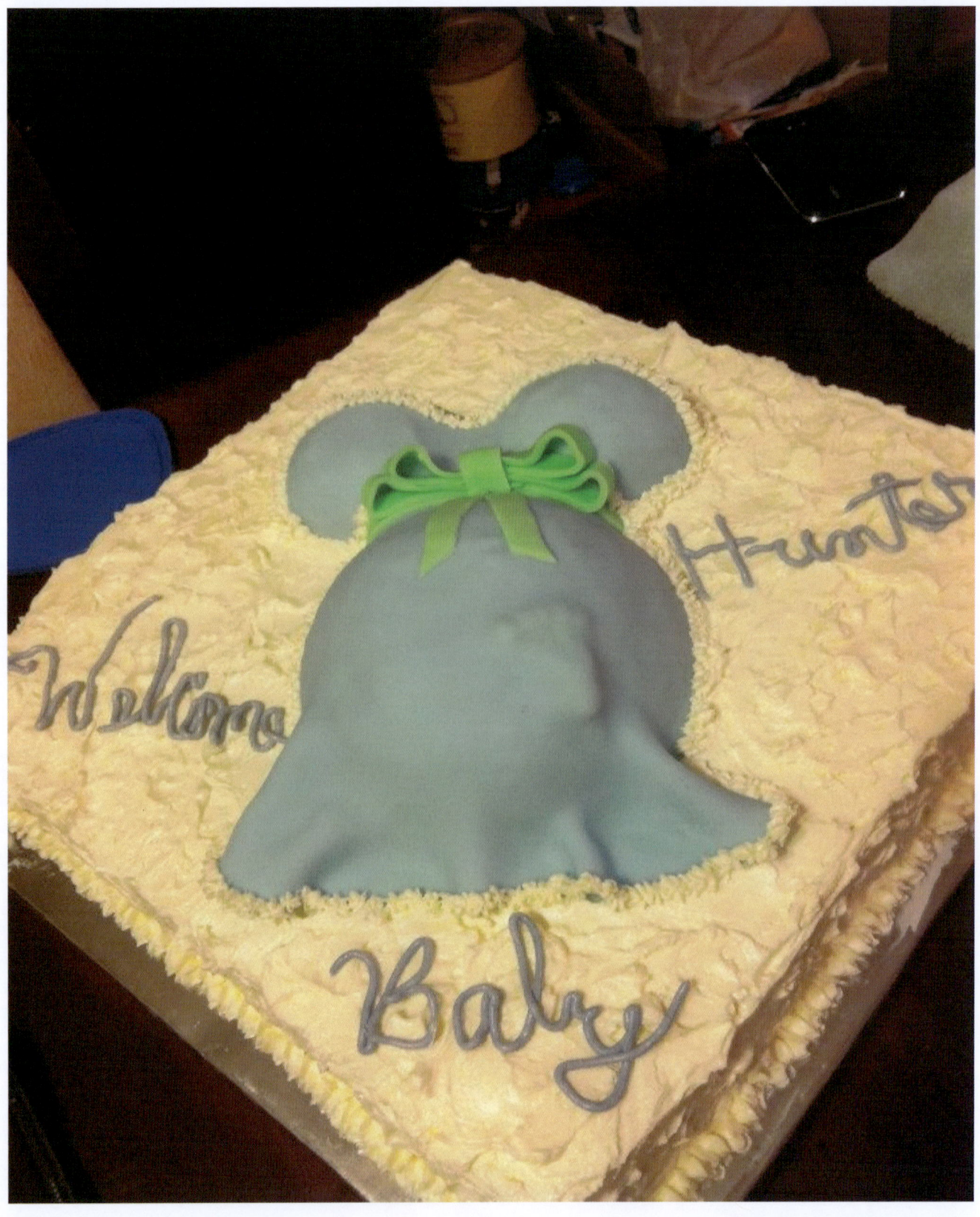

Homes

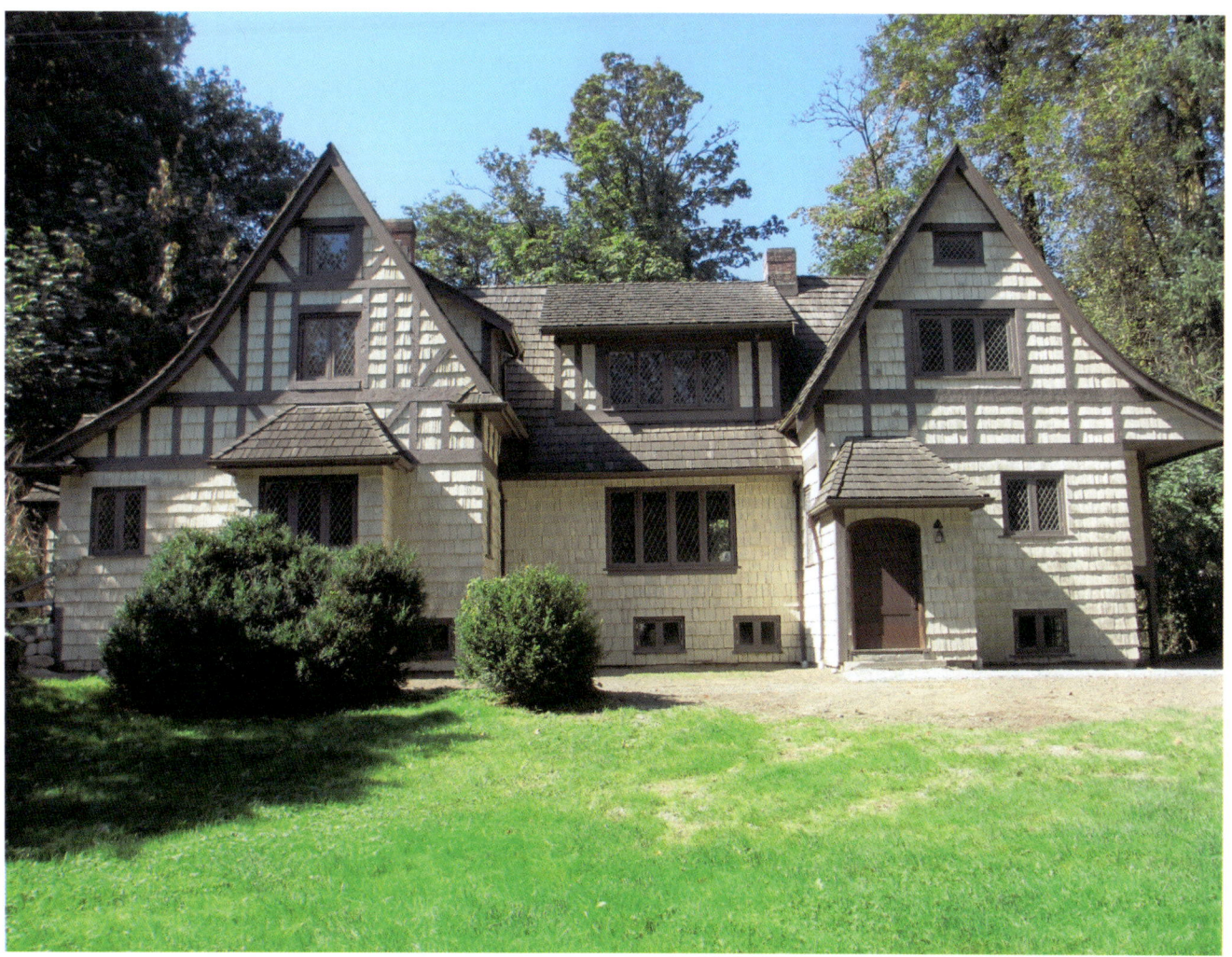

xc

1. What do you like about this house?

2. What do you dislike?

3. How much do you think it costs?

4. Would you consider purchasing it?

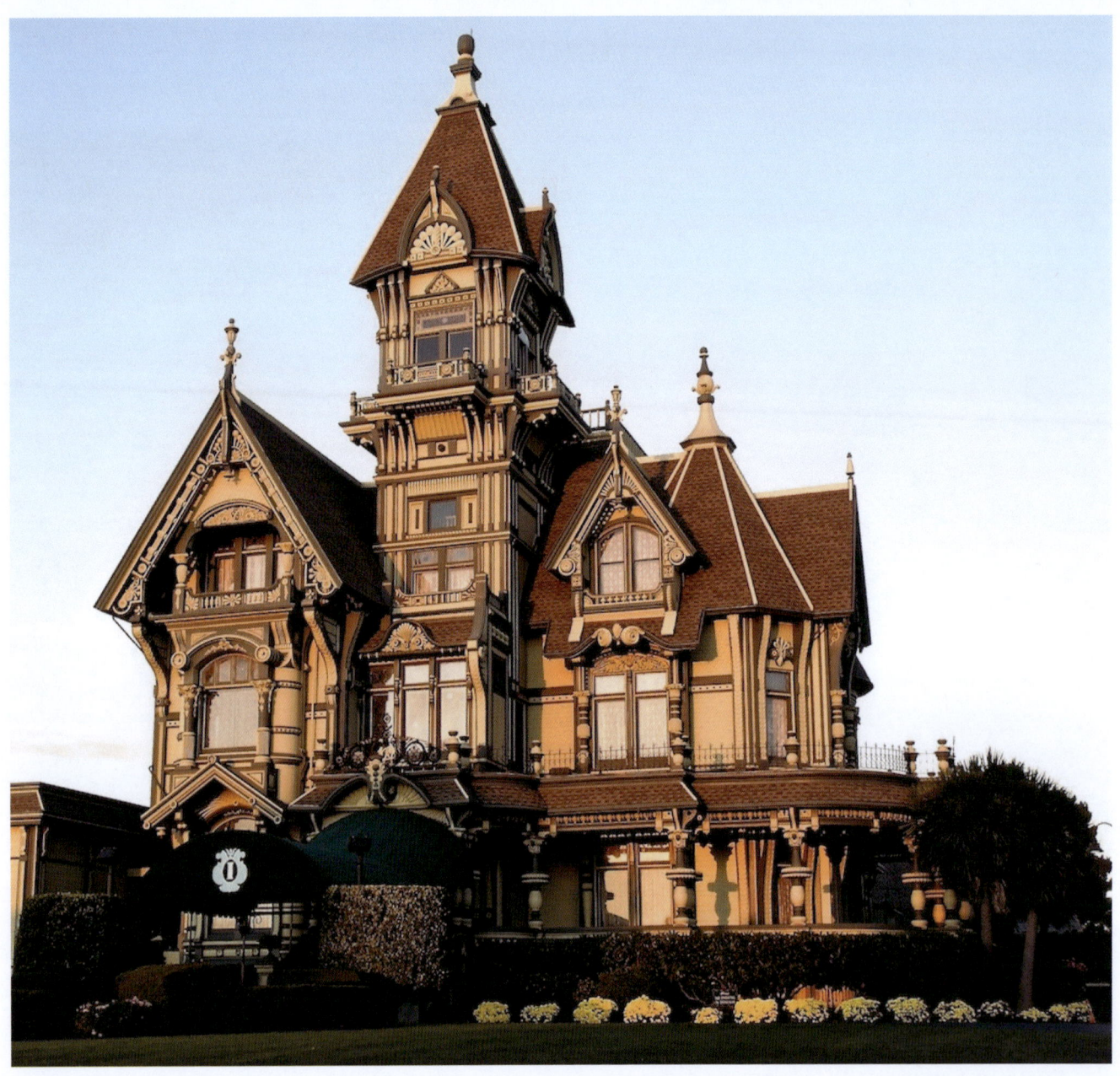

xci

1.   How many square feet do you think this home is?

2.   What is an interesting feature?

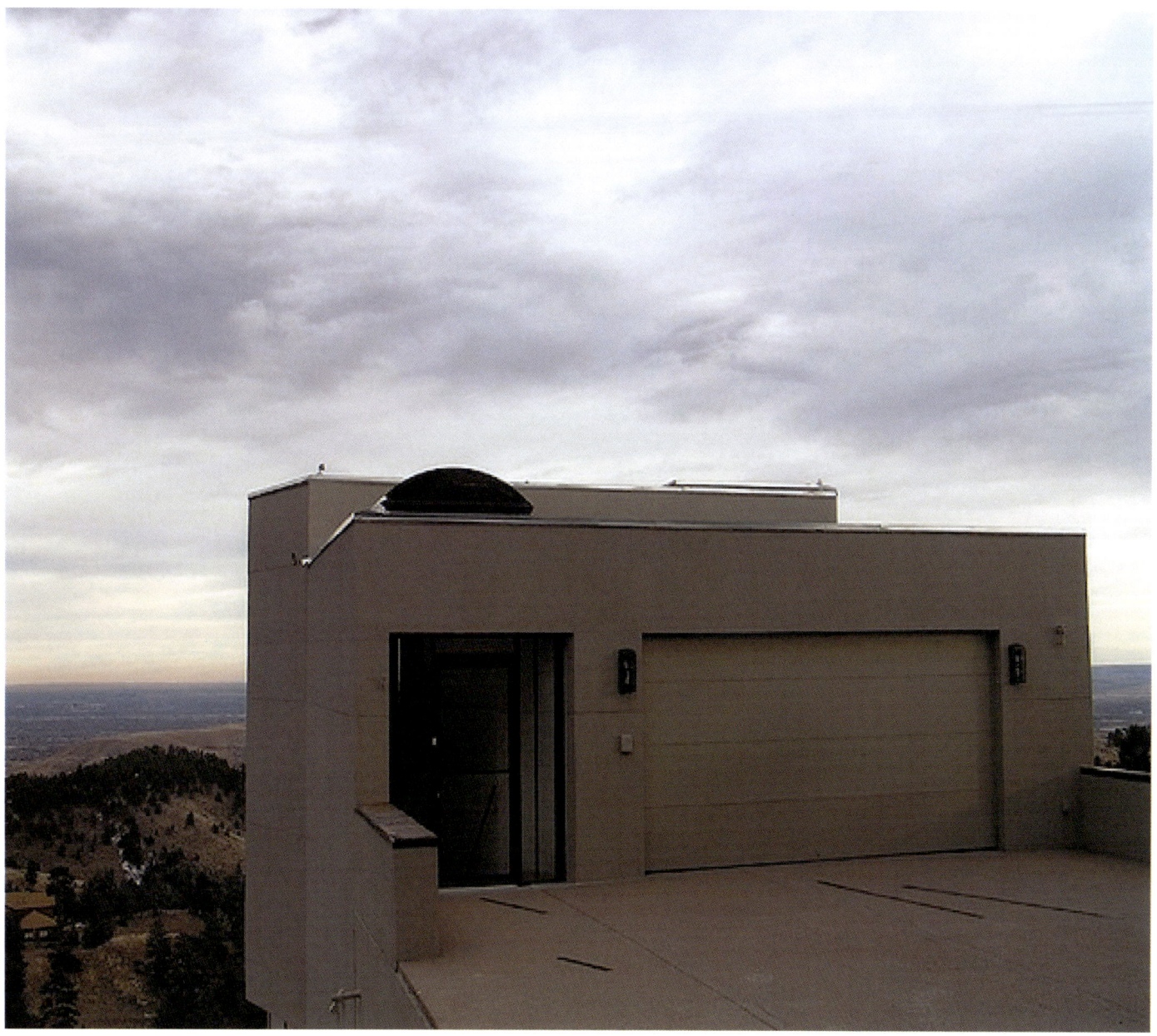

1. What style of home is this?

2. Do you like it?

3. Where is it located?

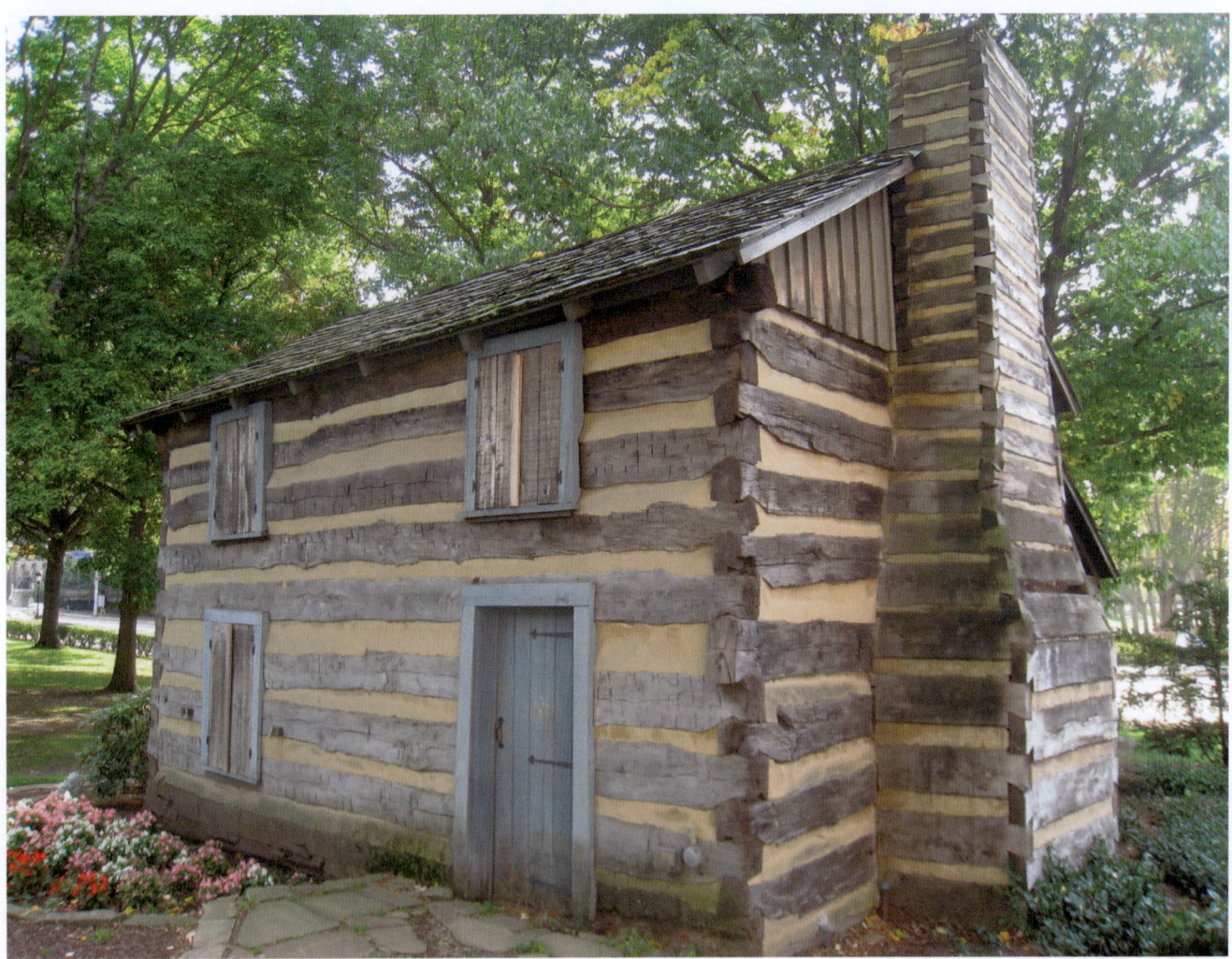

xciii

1.   What style of home is this?

2.   Do you think somebody lives in it? Why? Why not?

3.   What is unique about this home?

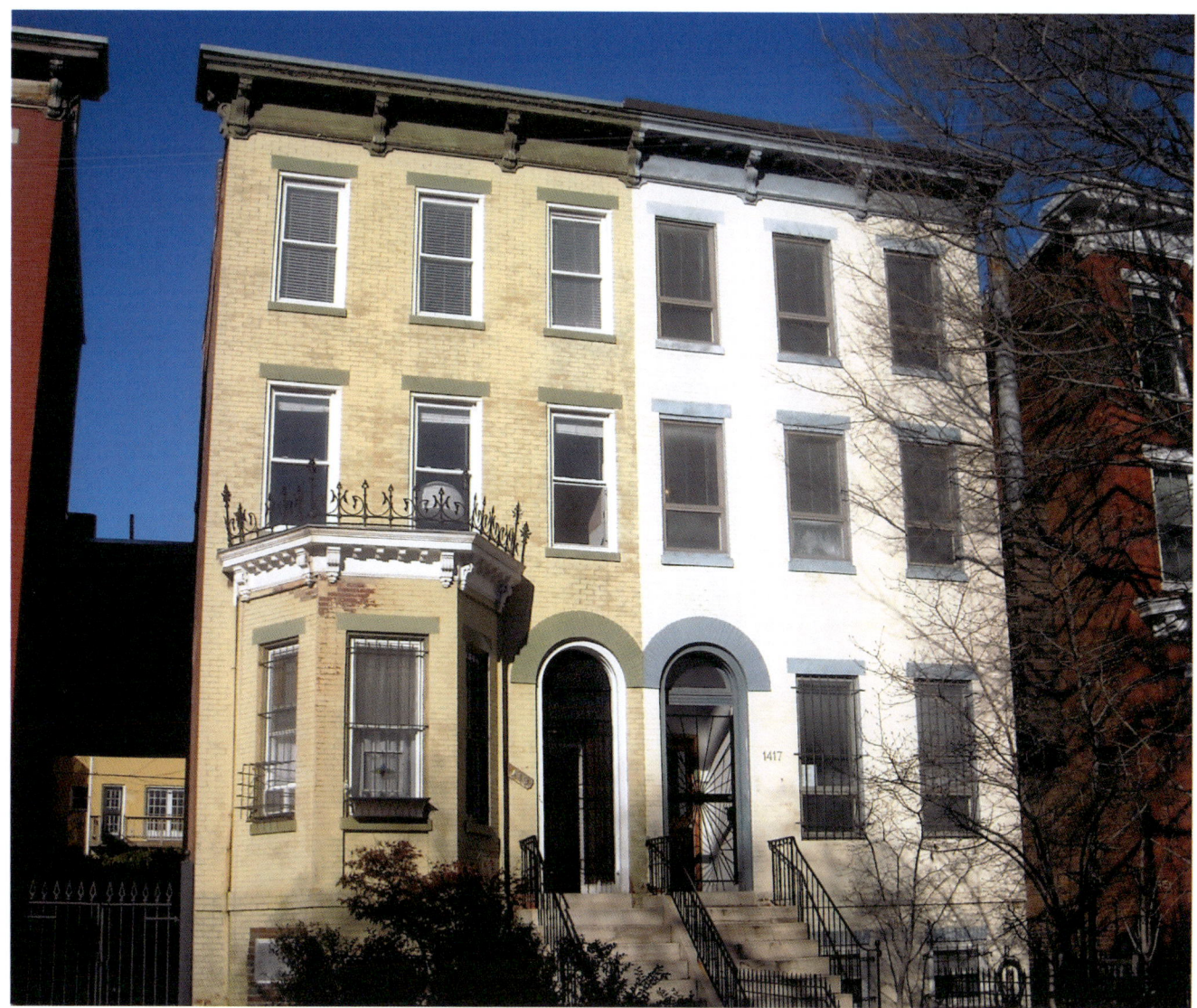

1.   Where is this home located?

2.   What type of home is this?

3.   How many stories do you think it is?

4.   Have you ever lived in a home like this?

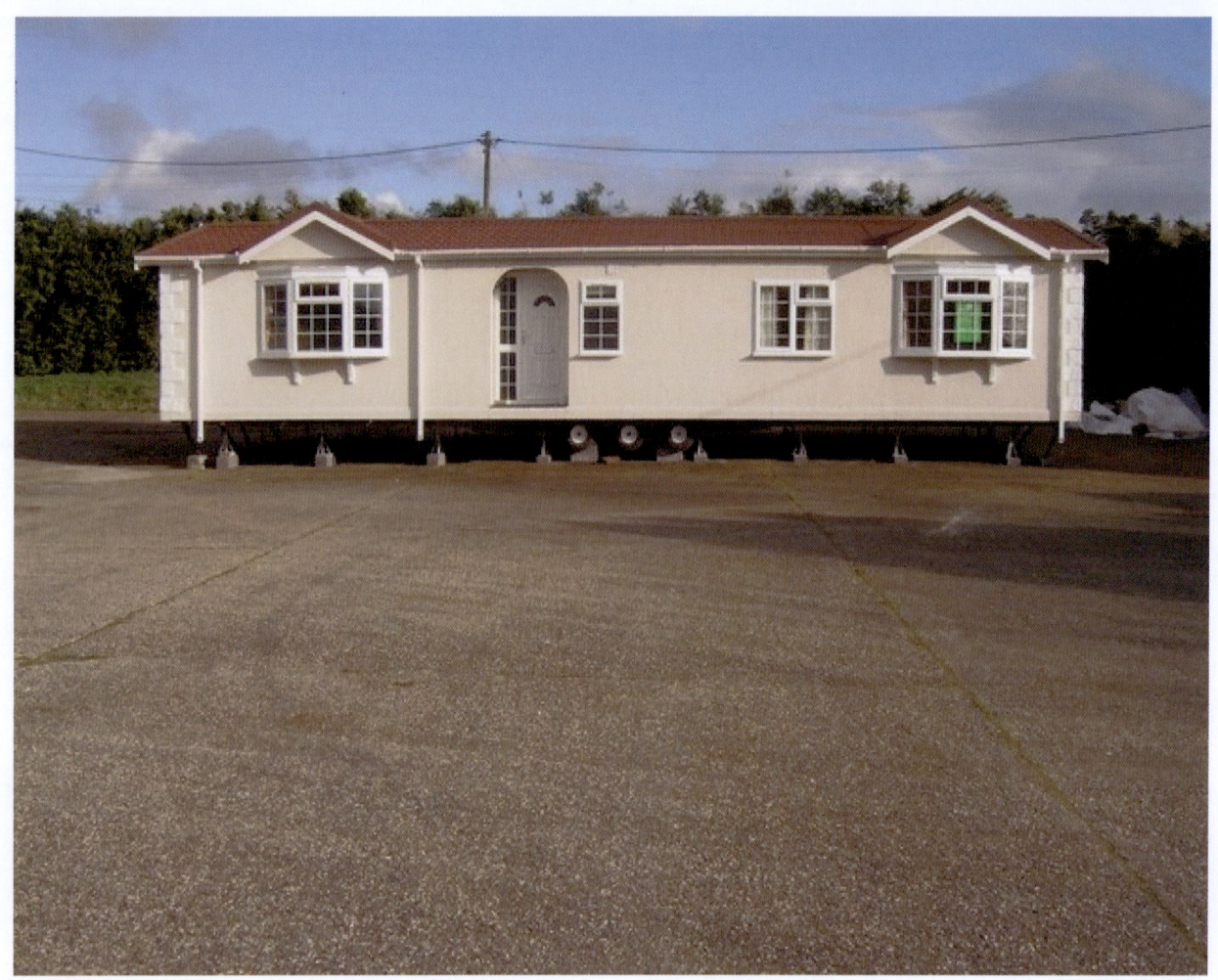

1.   What style of home is this?

2.   How much do you think it costs?

3.   What is unique about this style of home?

4.   What is this home resting on?

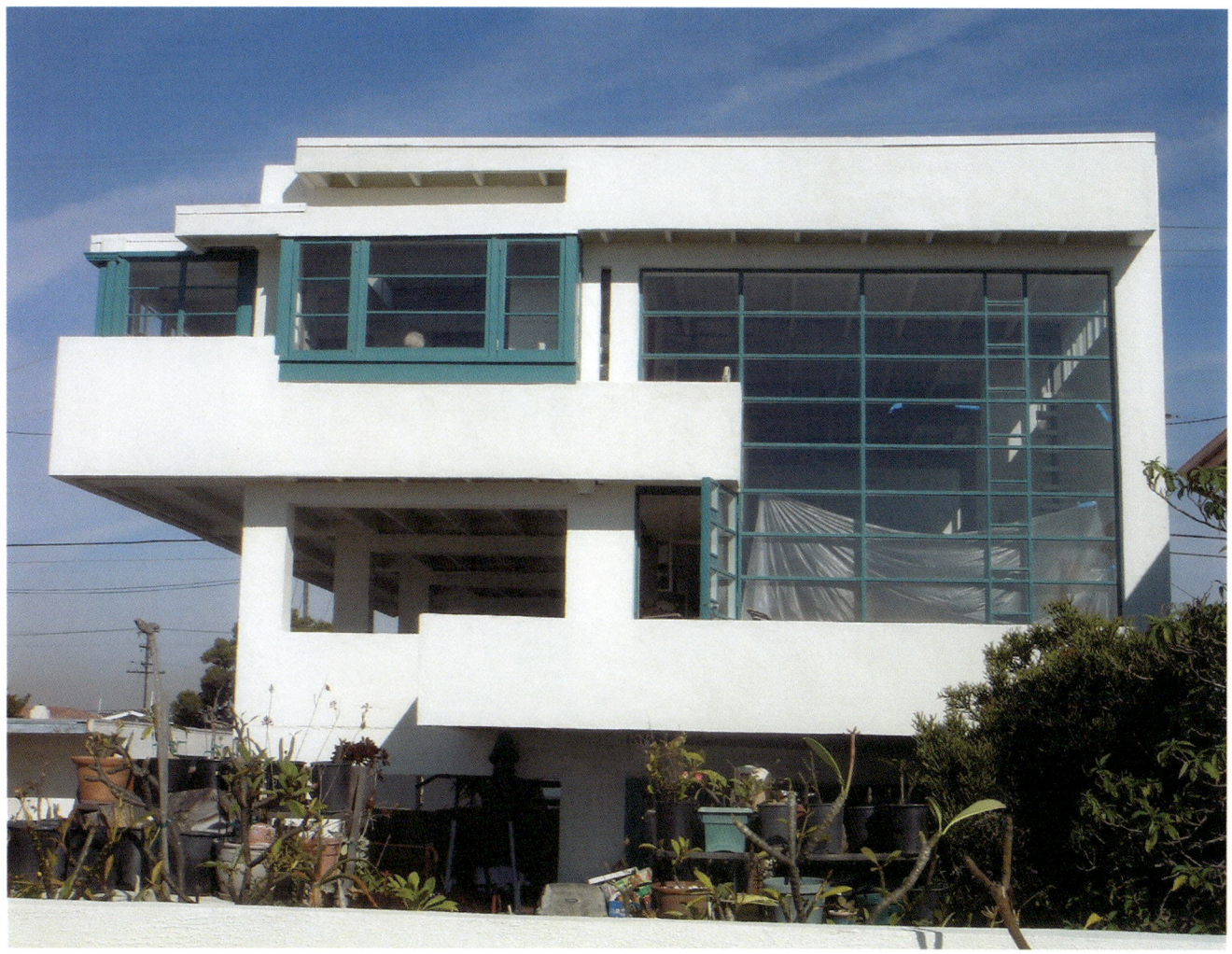

xcvi

1. What style of home is this?

2. Where do you think it is located? Why?

3. Would you like to live here? Why? Why Not?

4. What do you like about it?

5. What do you dislike?

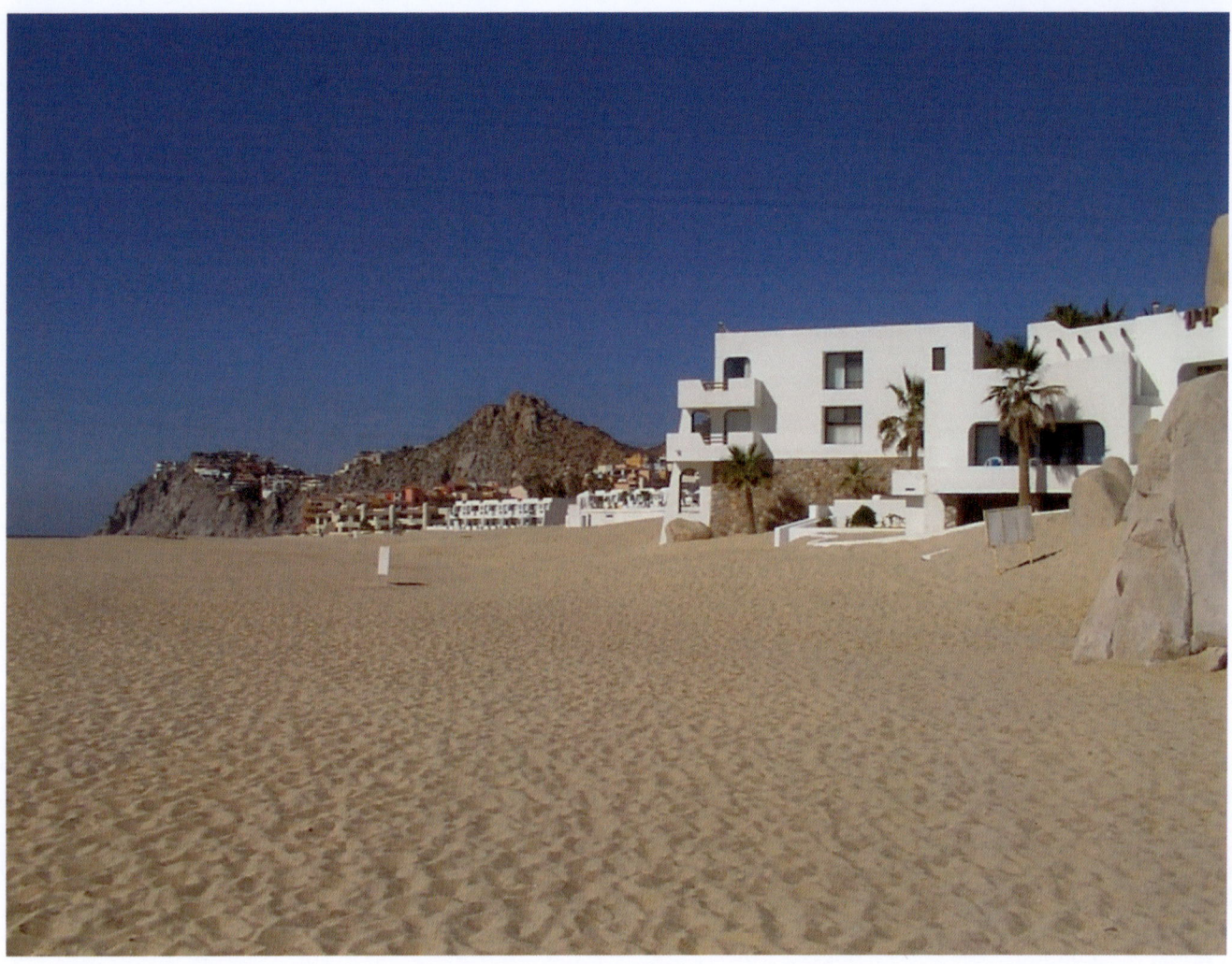

xcvii

1. Have you ever stayed at a place like this? Where? When?

2. Would you like to live here?

3. What are some possible risks of living here?

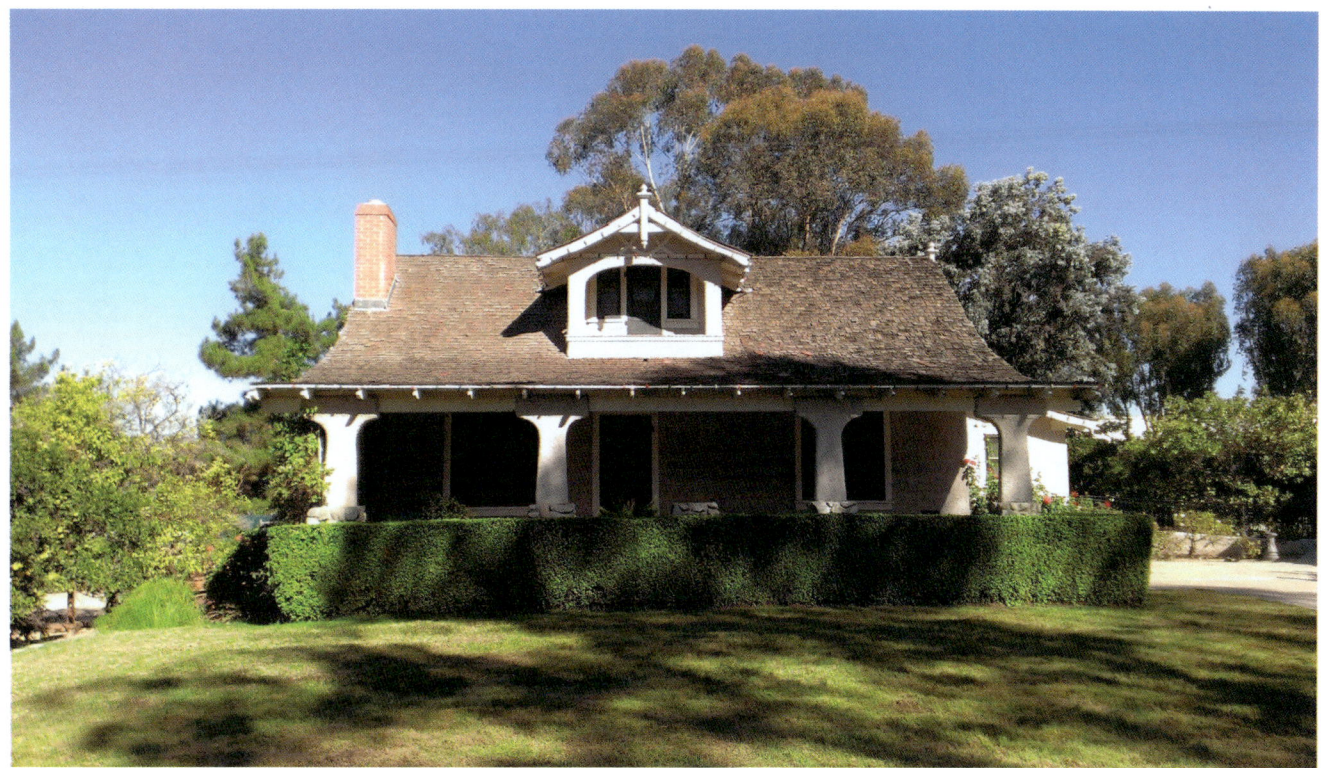

xcviii

1. What style of home is this?

2. What do you like about it?

3. What do you dislike?

4. Where do you think it is located?

5. How much do you think it costs?

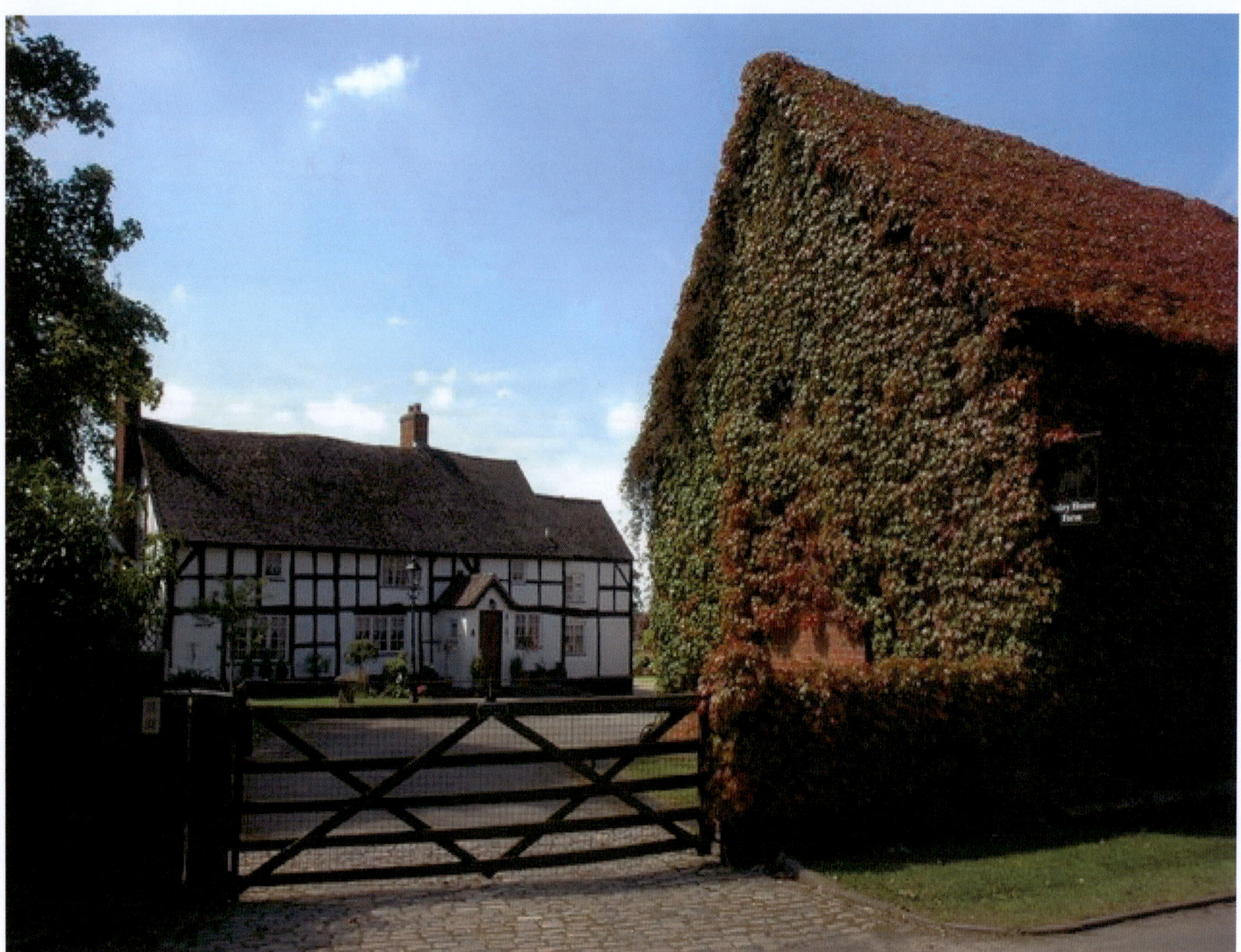

1. What style home is this?

2. Where is it located?

3. What type of building is next to it?

4. Of all the homes, which one is your favorite? Why?

Describing Photographs

conversation starters

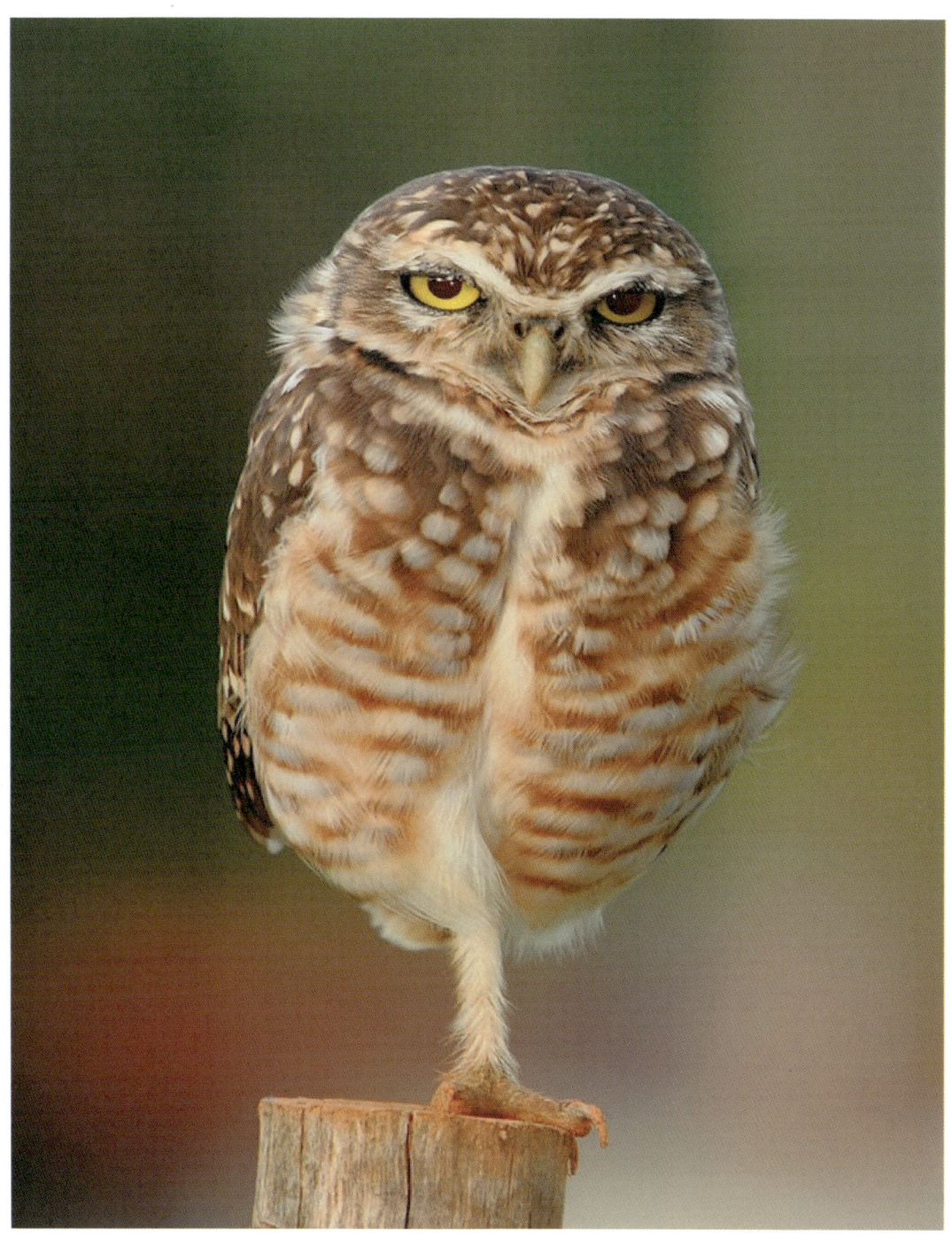

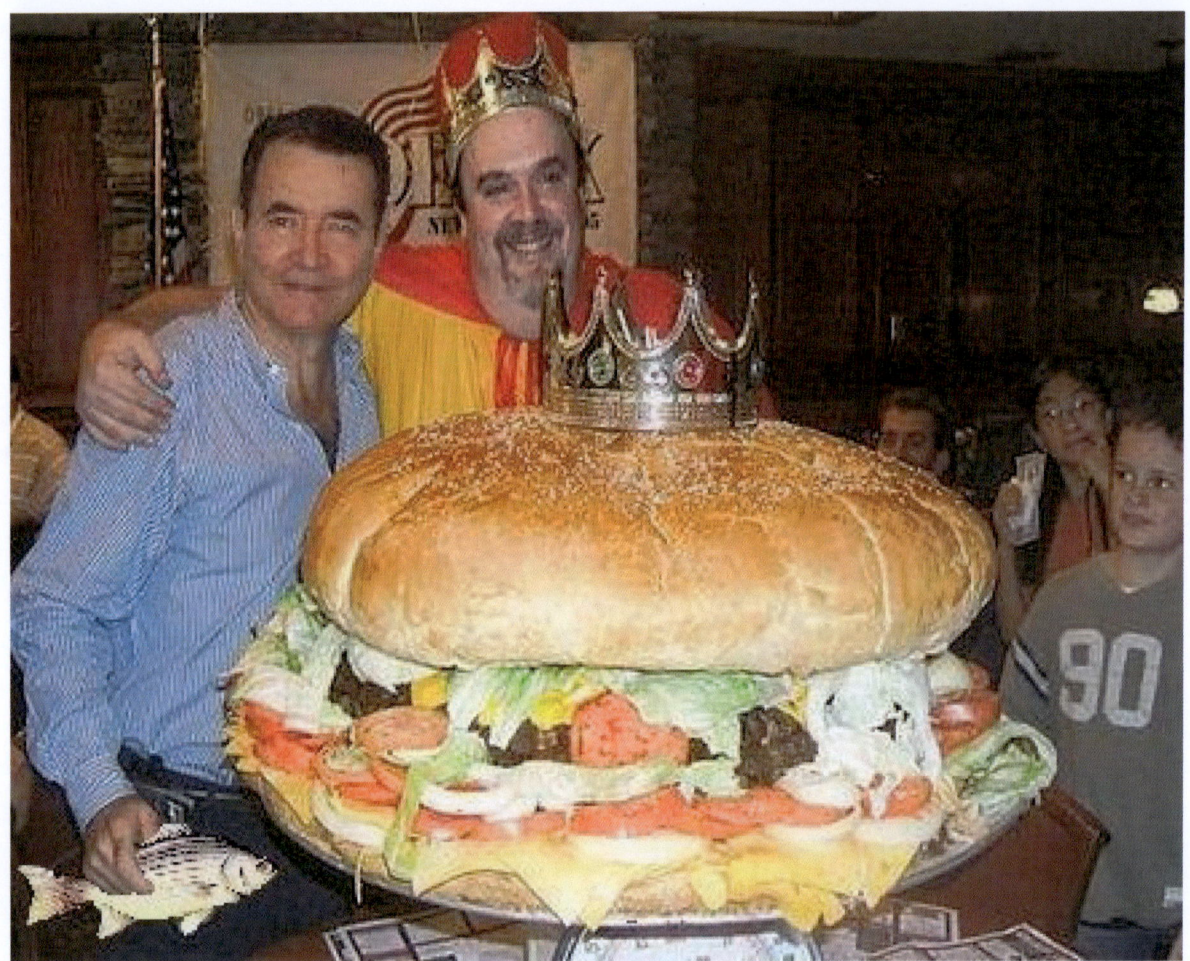

ci

1. Describe the photograph.

2. How much money would you want to eat the entire burger?

3. Have you ever participated in an eating contest?

4. What is your favorite food?

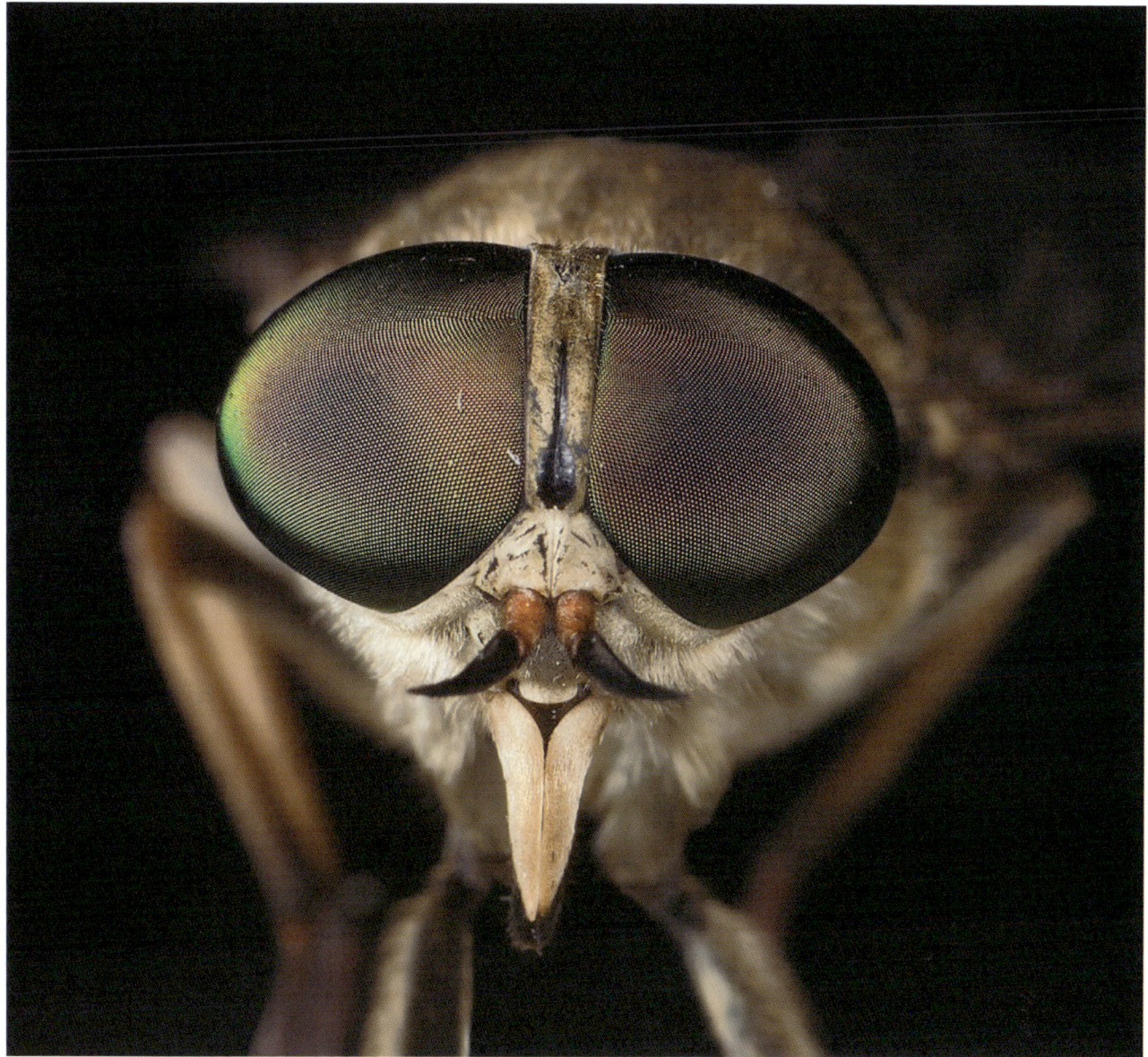

cii

1. What do you think this is?

2. What is the strangest insect you have ever seen?

3. Do you know anyone who is allergic to insects?

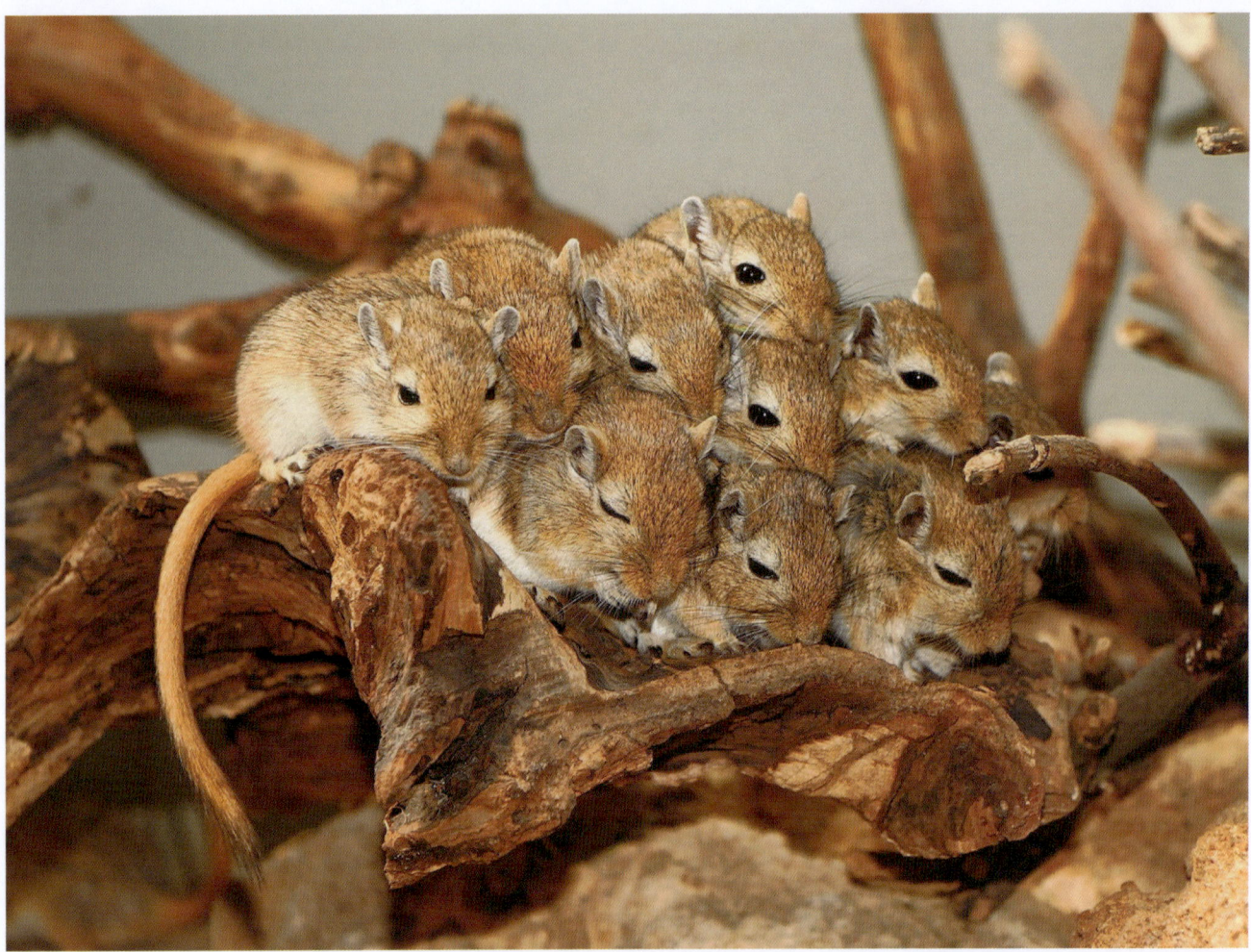

ciii

1. Describe the photograph.

2. What would you do if you saw them?

3. If you have had mice in your house, what did you do?

4. What was the smallest pet you ever owned?

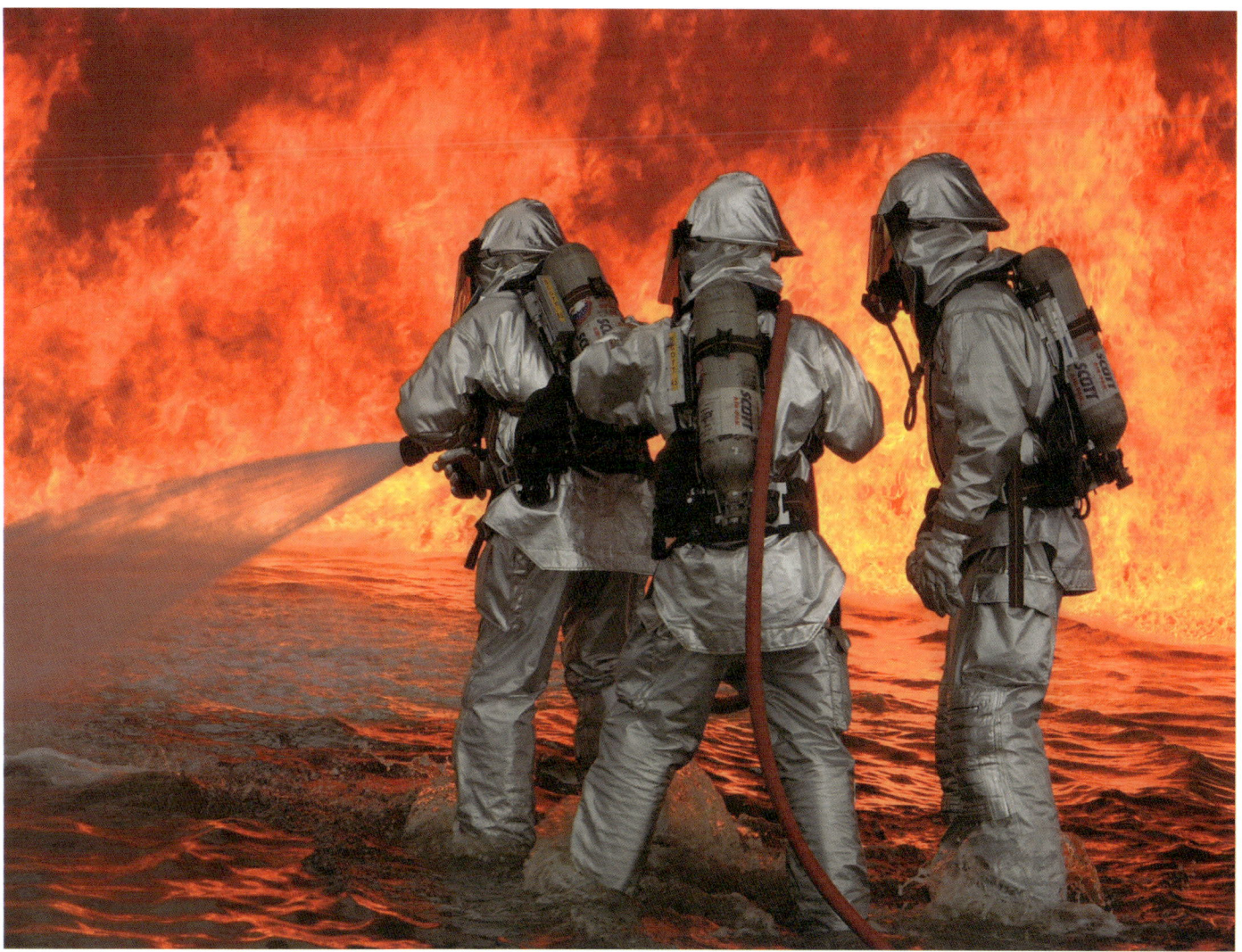

civ

1. Describe the photograph.

2. What is happening?

3. Why are they wearing masks?

4. What would you do in this situation?

5. Describe an experience you or someone you know has had with fire.

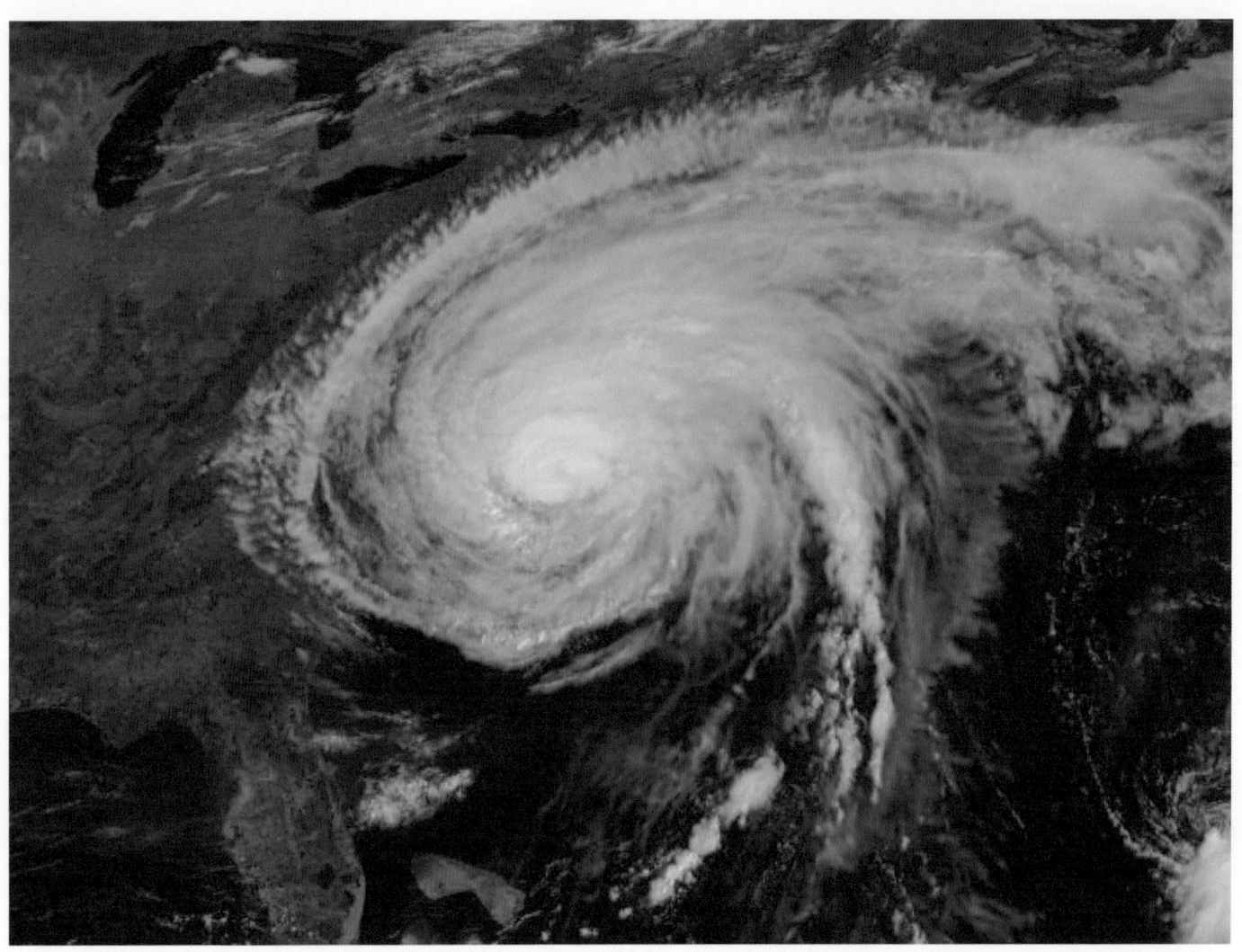

cv

1. Describe the photograph.

2. Where is this storm?

3. Describe your experience with hurricanes.

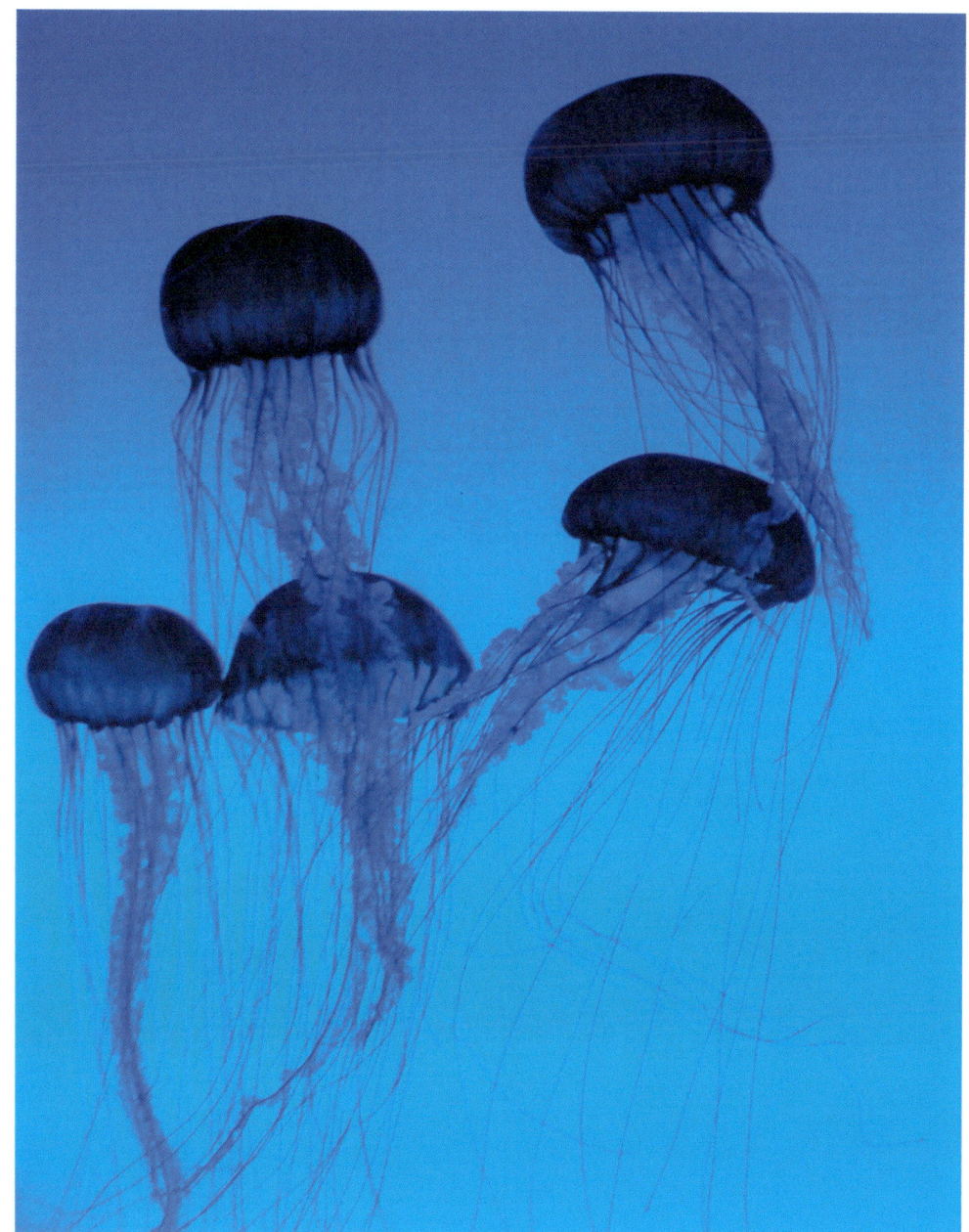

1. Describe the photograph using at least 4 adjectives.

2. Where is this?

3. How many are there?

4. Describe an encounter that you have had with a jelly fish.

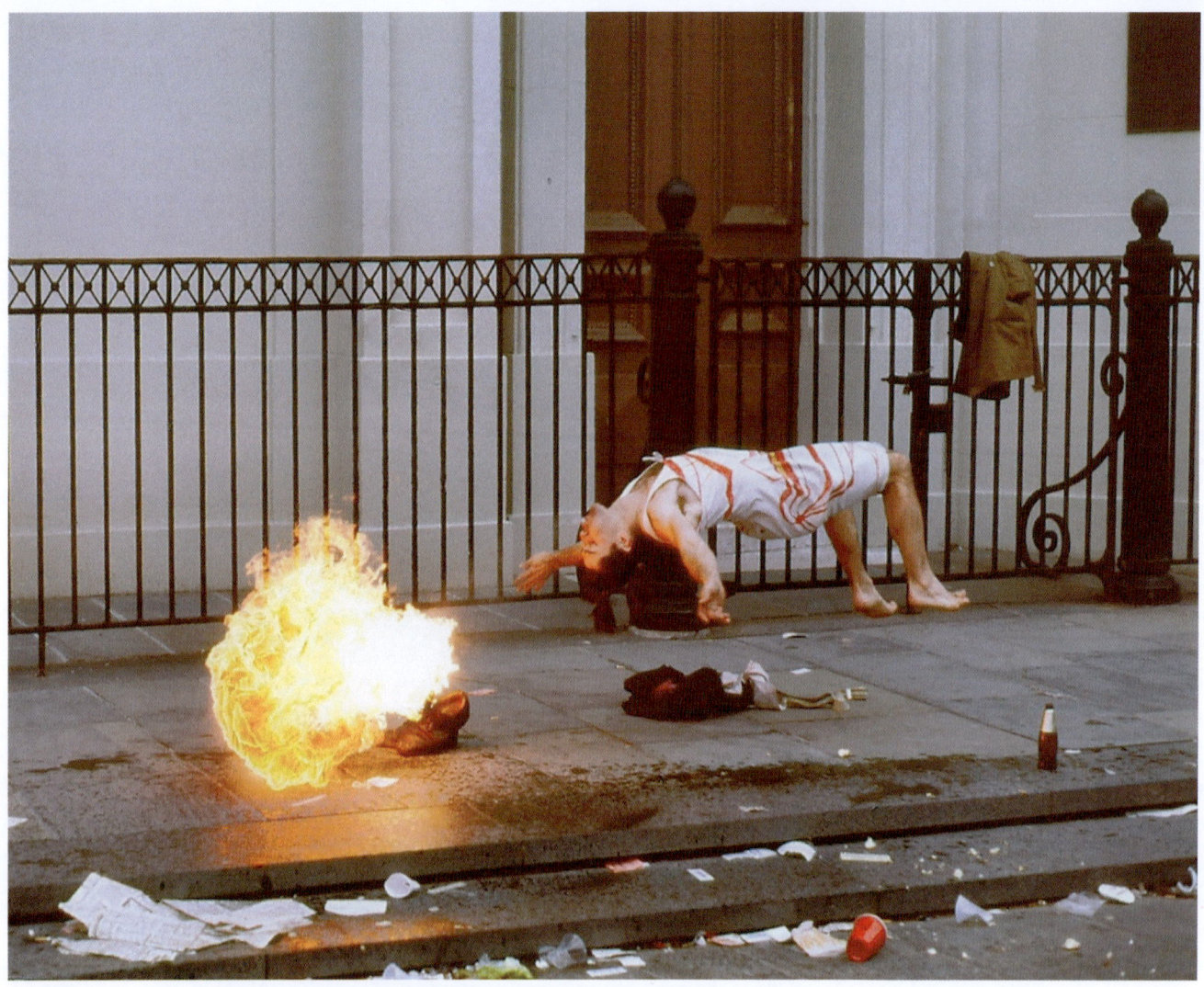

cvii

1. What is this man doing?

2. Would you stay to watch if you were there? Why? Why not?

3. Do you think he is flipping or levitating?

4. Describe the sidewalk and street.

5. Have you ever seen anything remotely like this?

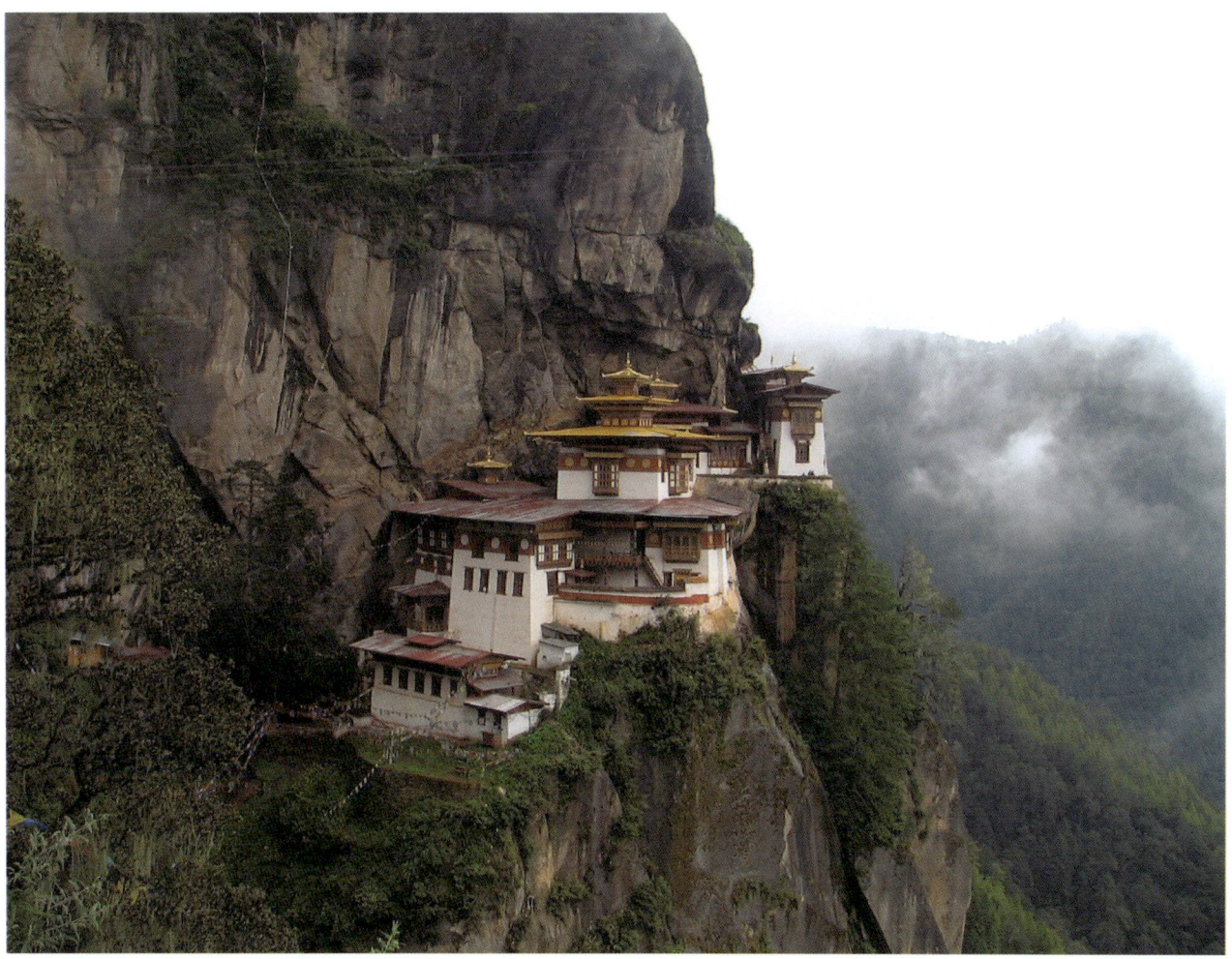

cviii

1.   Describe the photograph.

2.   Explain how they could have gotten the building materials there?

4.   What part of the world do you think this is? Why?

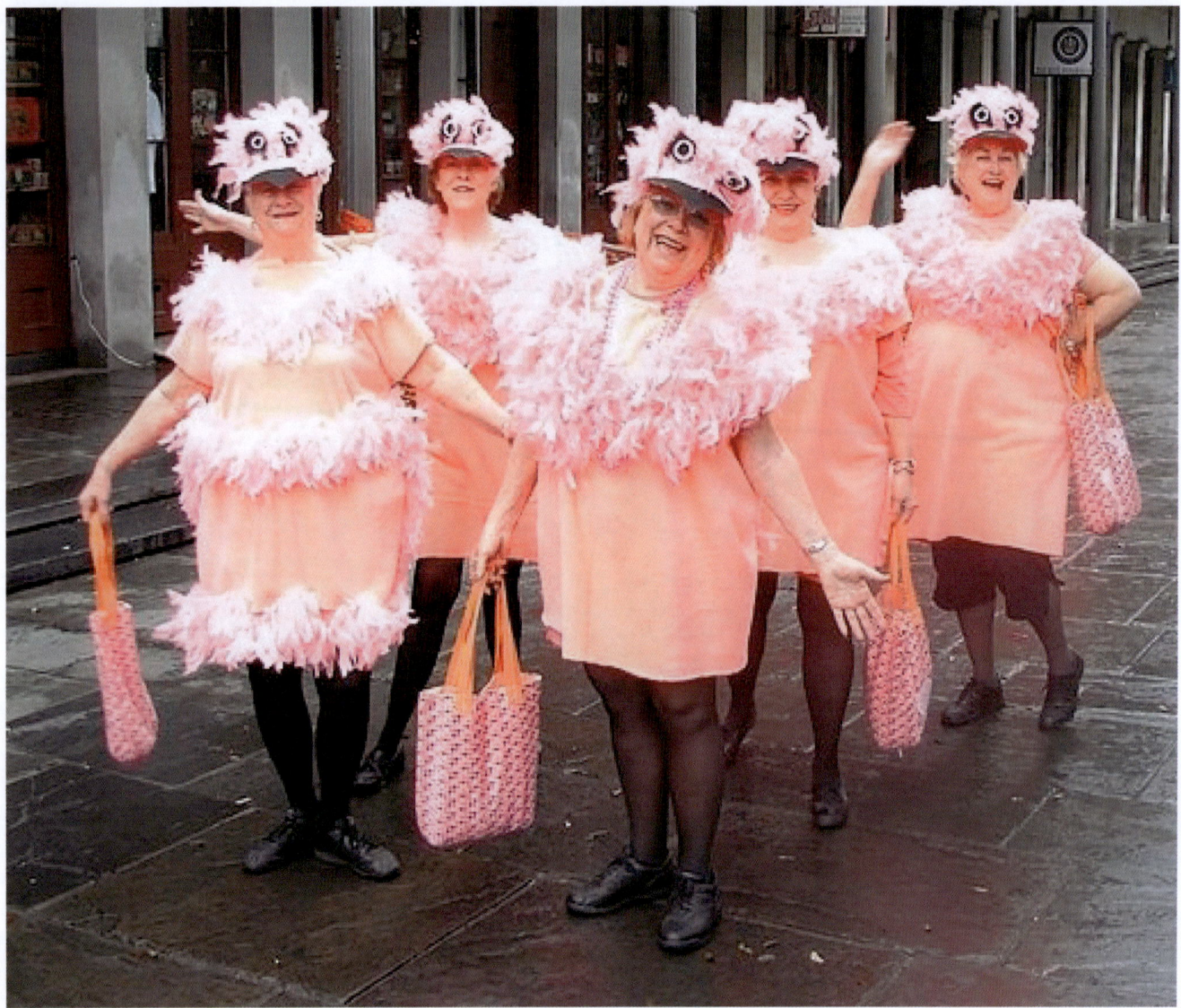

cix

1. Describe the photograph using at least 4 adjectives.

2. What makes the picture unique?

3. Why do you think they dressed up?

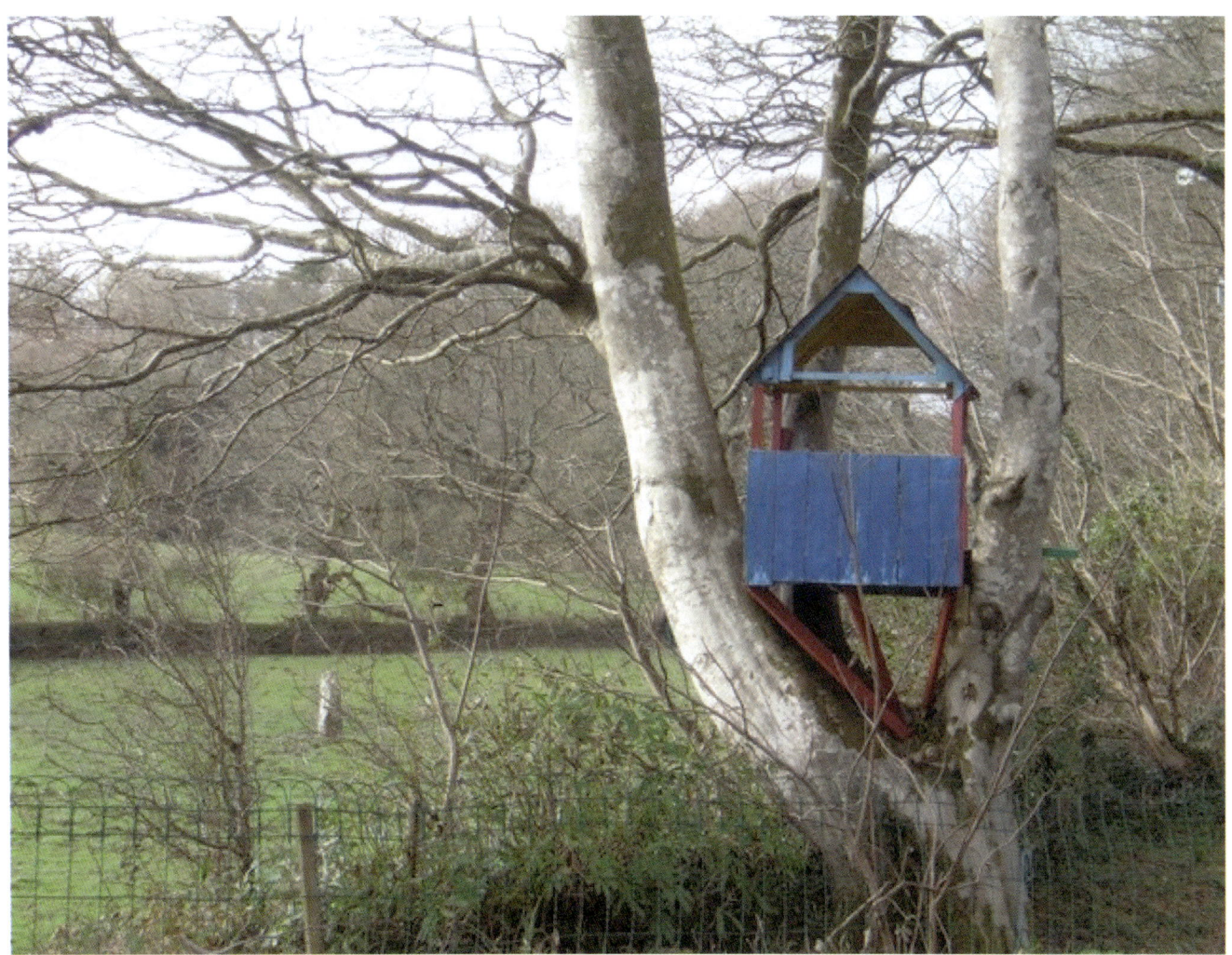

cx

1. Describe the photograph.

2. Who would use this?

3. What did you play with outdoors when you were a kid?

4. What time of year is it?

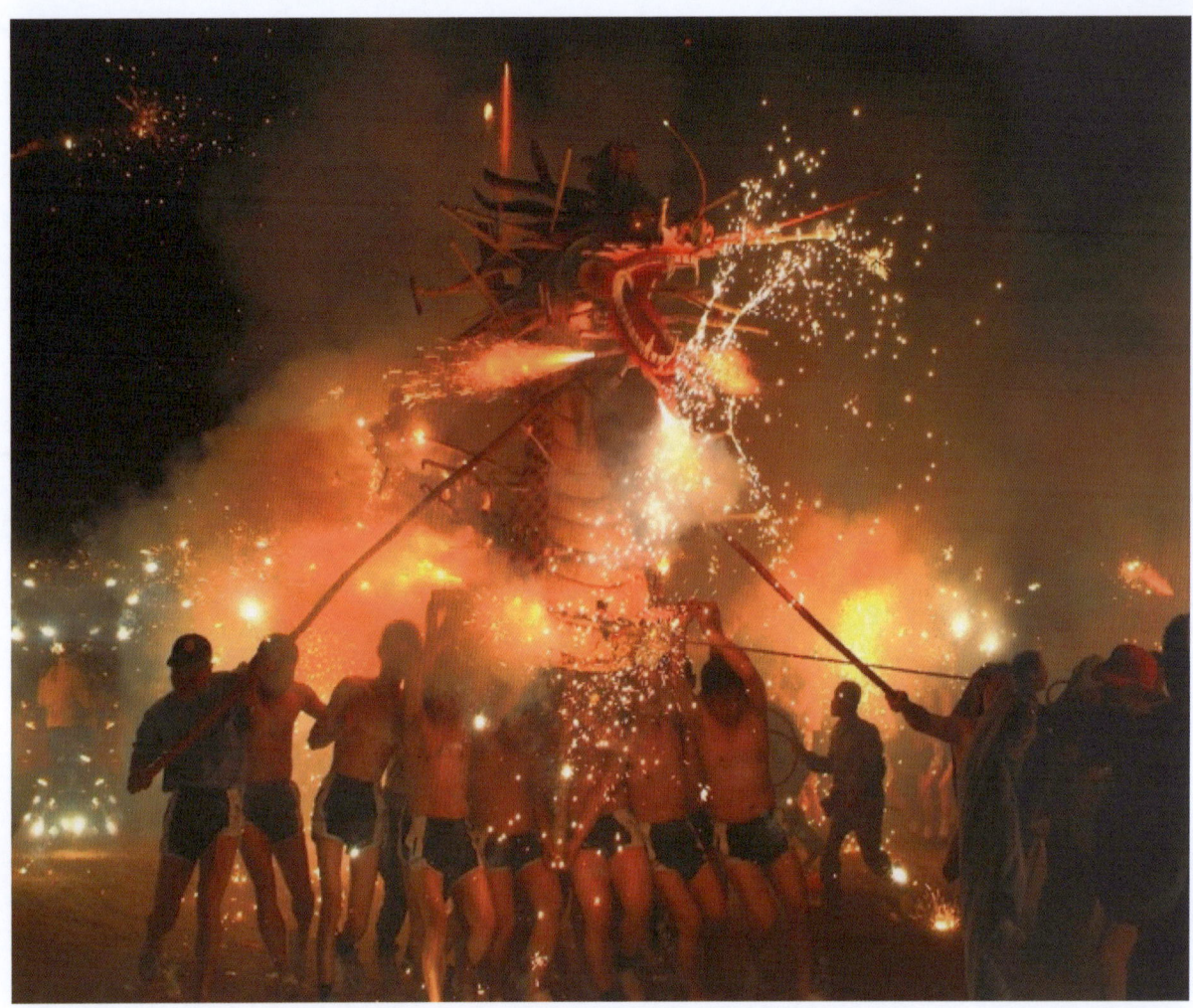

1. Describe the photograph.

2. Have you ever seen a similar performance?

3. Where do you think this photo was taken?

4. What celebration do you think it is for?

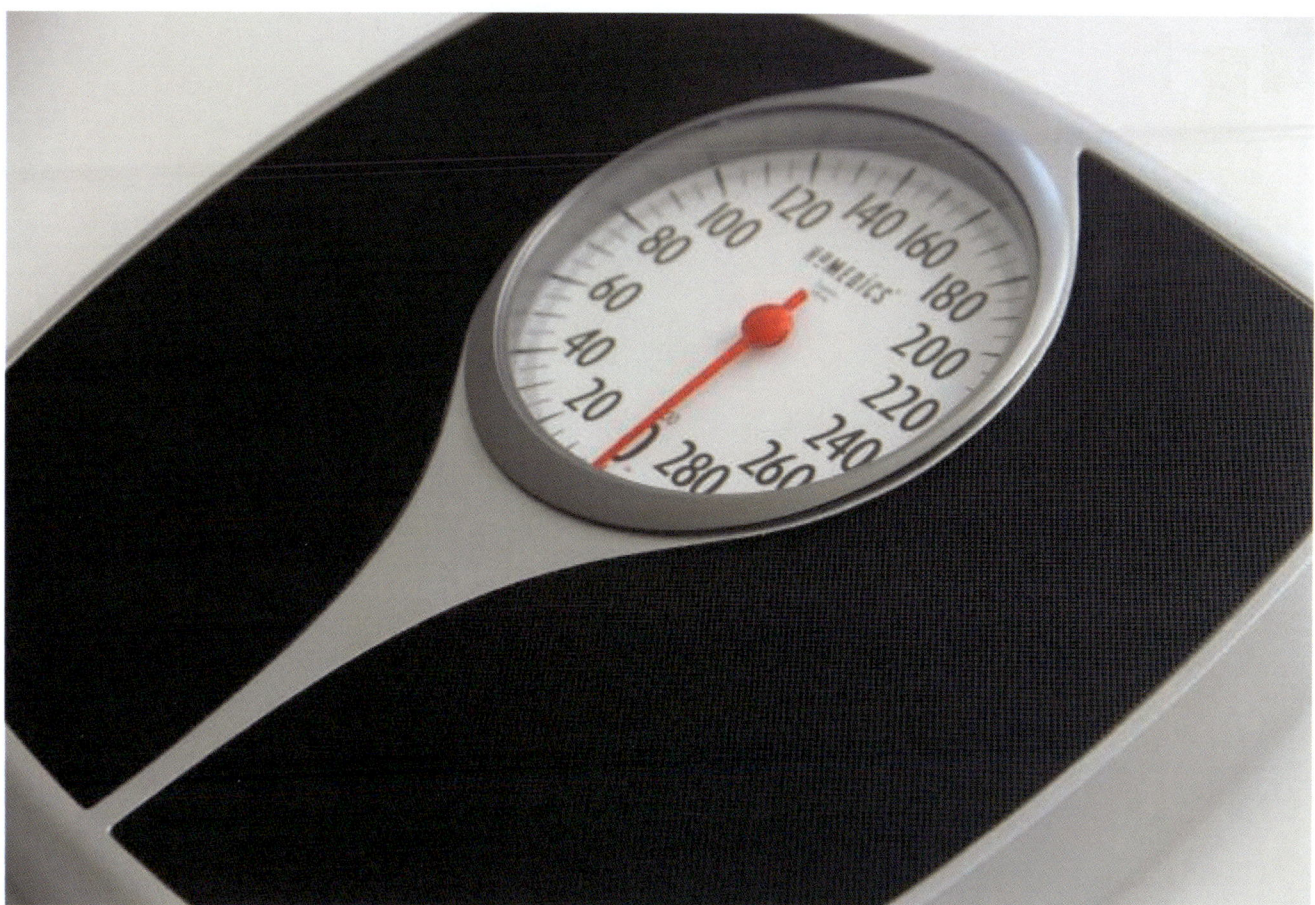

1. Do people like to get on one of these?

2. When you diet, what do you do to loose weight?

3. What type of exercise do you prefer?

4. Have ever lost a great deal of weight?

5. What is your dream weight?

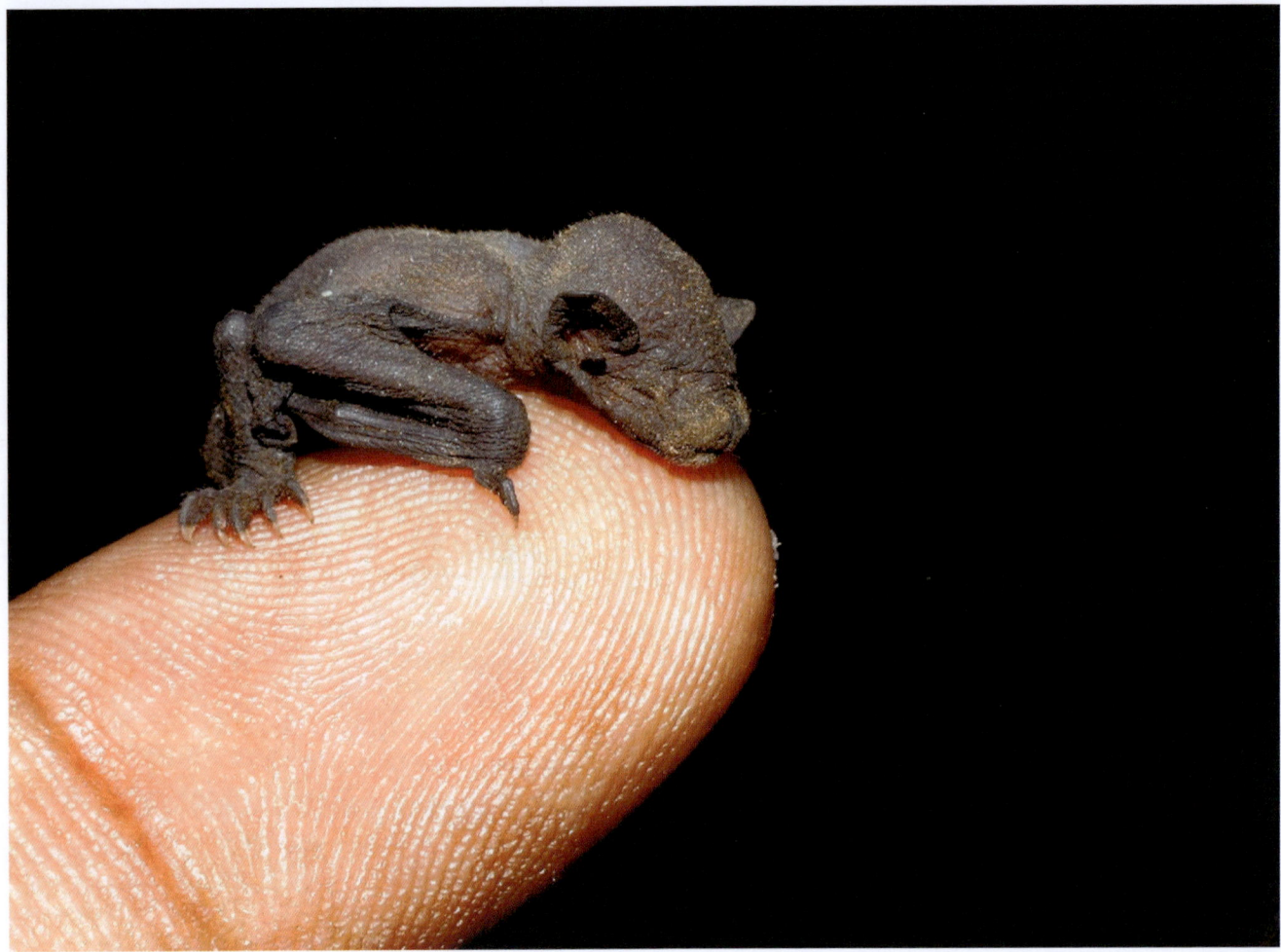

1. What do you think this is?

2. Describe the photograph?

3. It is a newborn bat. Would you hold it?

4. Do you think it is scary or cute?

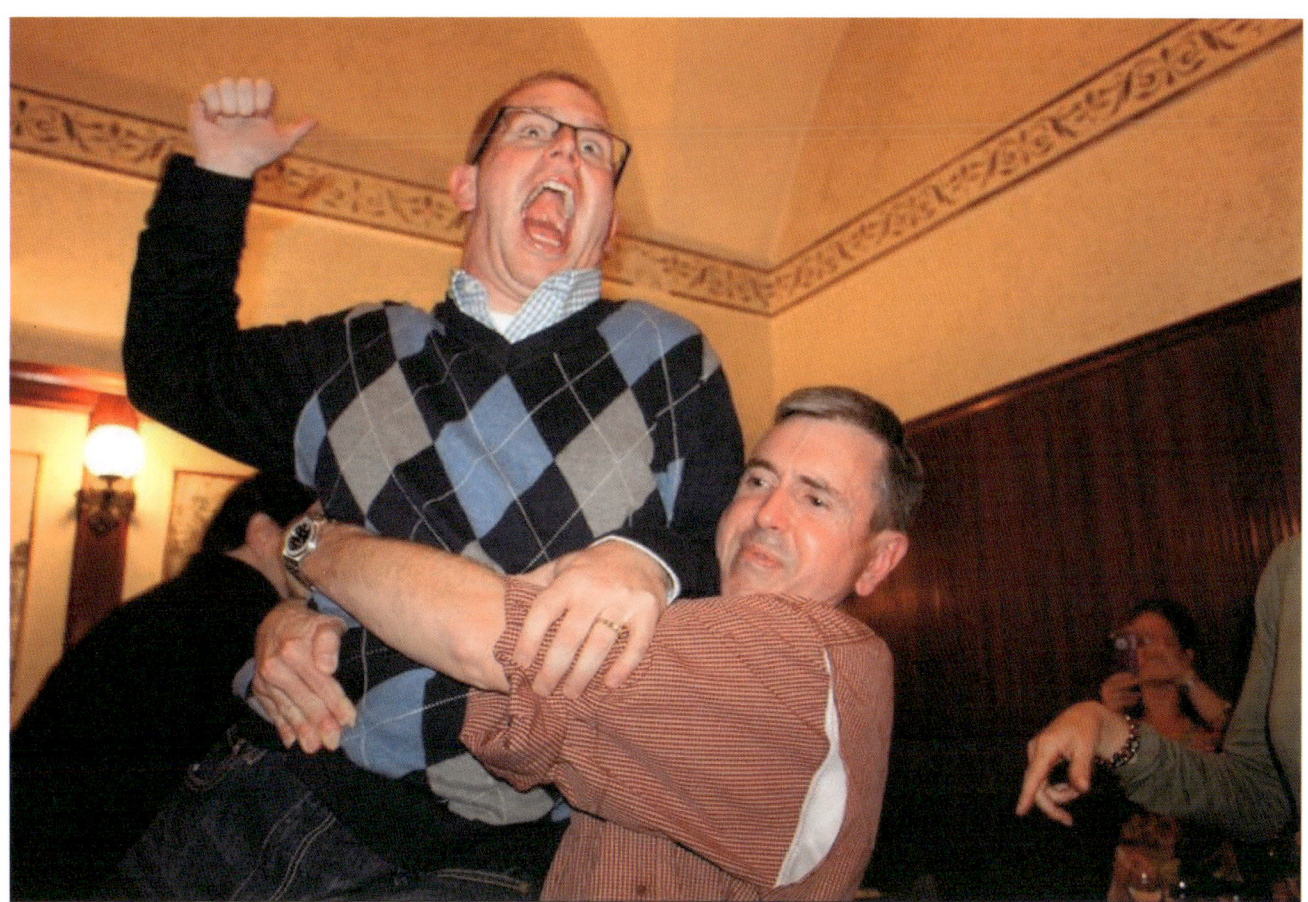

cxiv

1. Describe what is happening.

2. What do you think made him act like this?

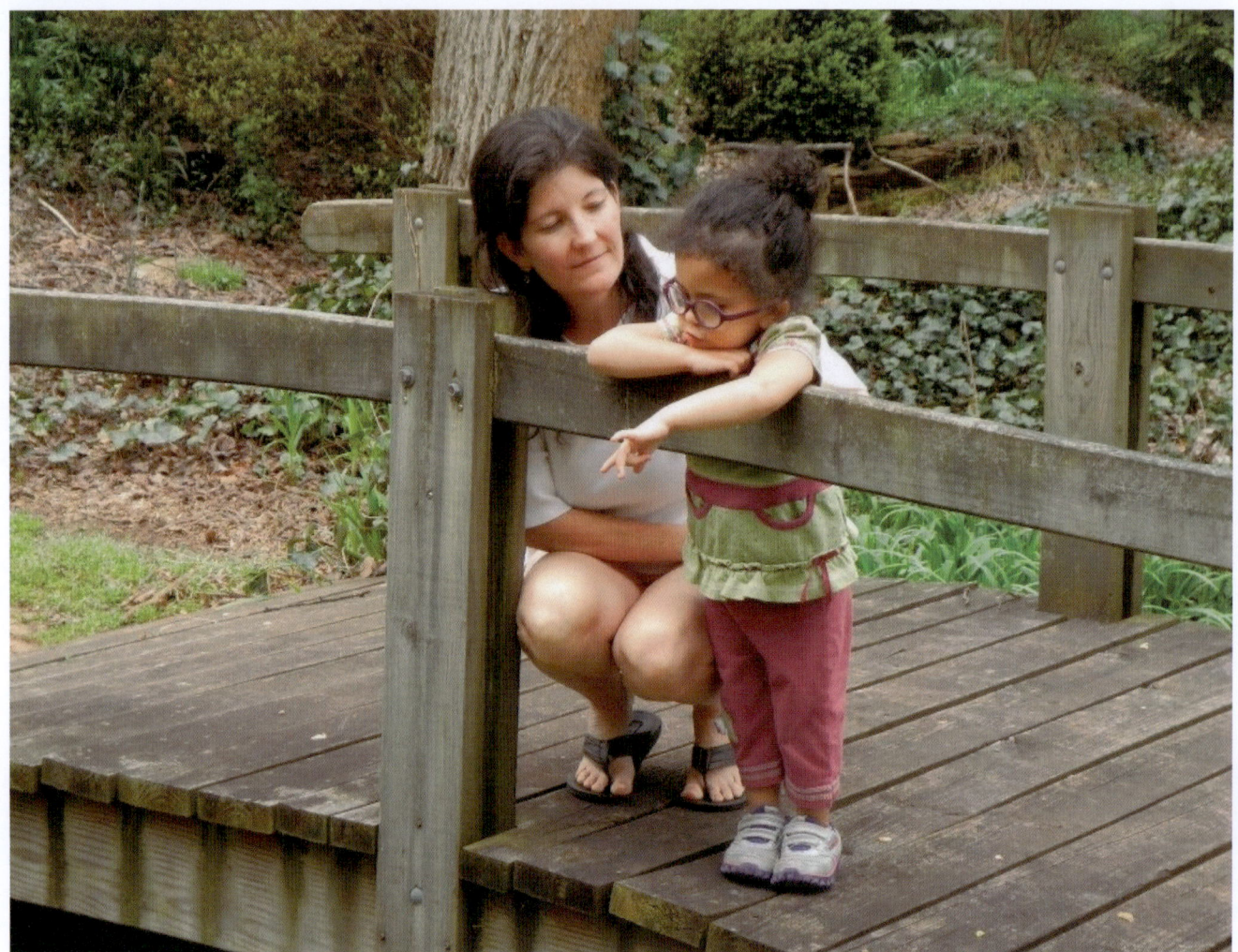

cxv

1.   Where are they?

2.   What do you think their relationship is?

3.   How does the mother feel about her daughter?

4.   What do you think the little girl is looking at?

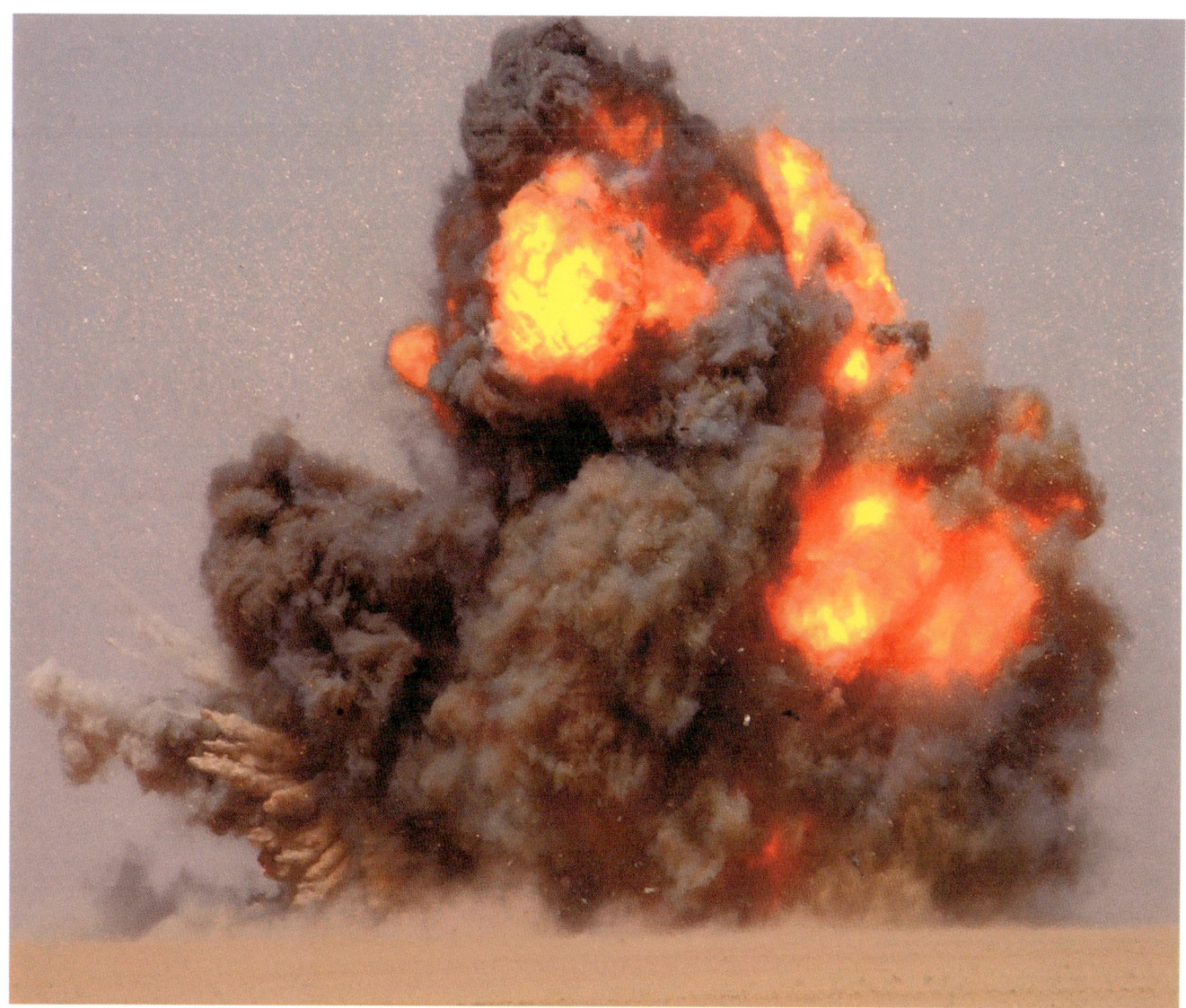

cxvi

1.	What happened?

2.	Where do you think this took place?

3.	Describe your or somebody you know's experience in the military?

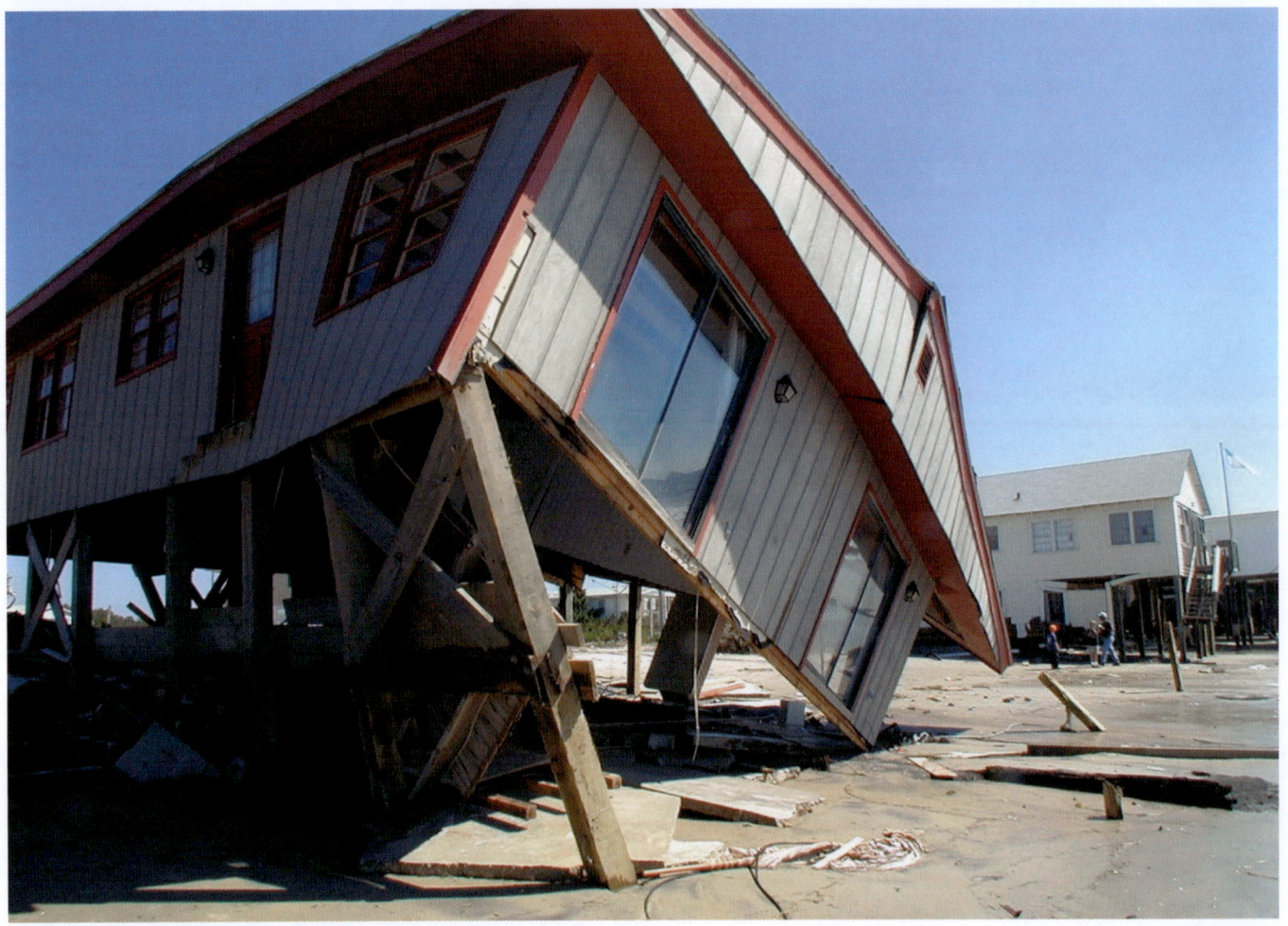

cxvii

1. What happened?

2. How do you think it happened?

3. Where is the house?

4. Do you think they can fix it? Why? Why not?

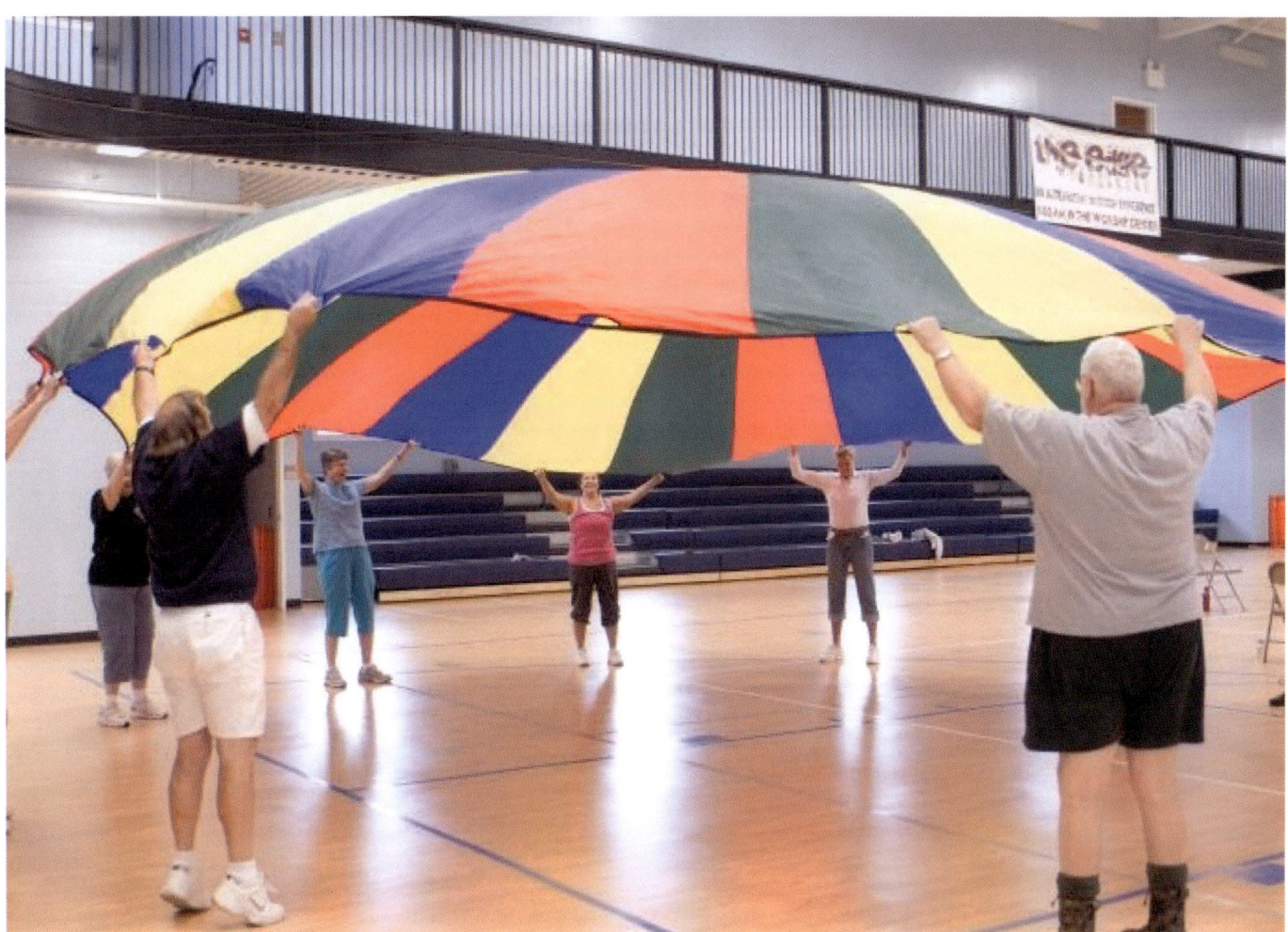

cxviii

1. What are they doing?

2. What kind of group do you think it is?

3. Where are they?

4. About how old do you think the participants are?

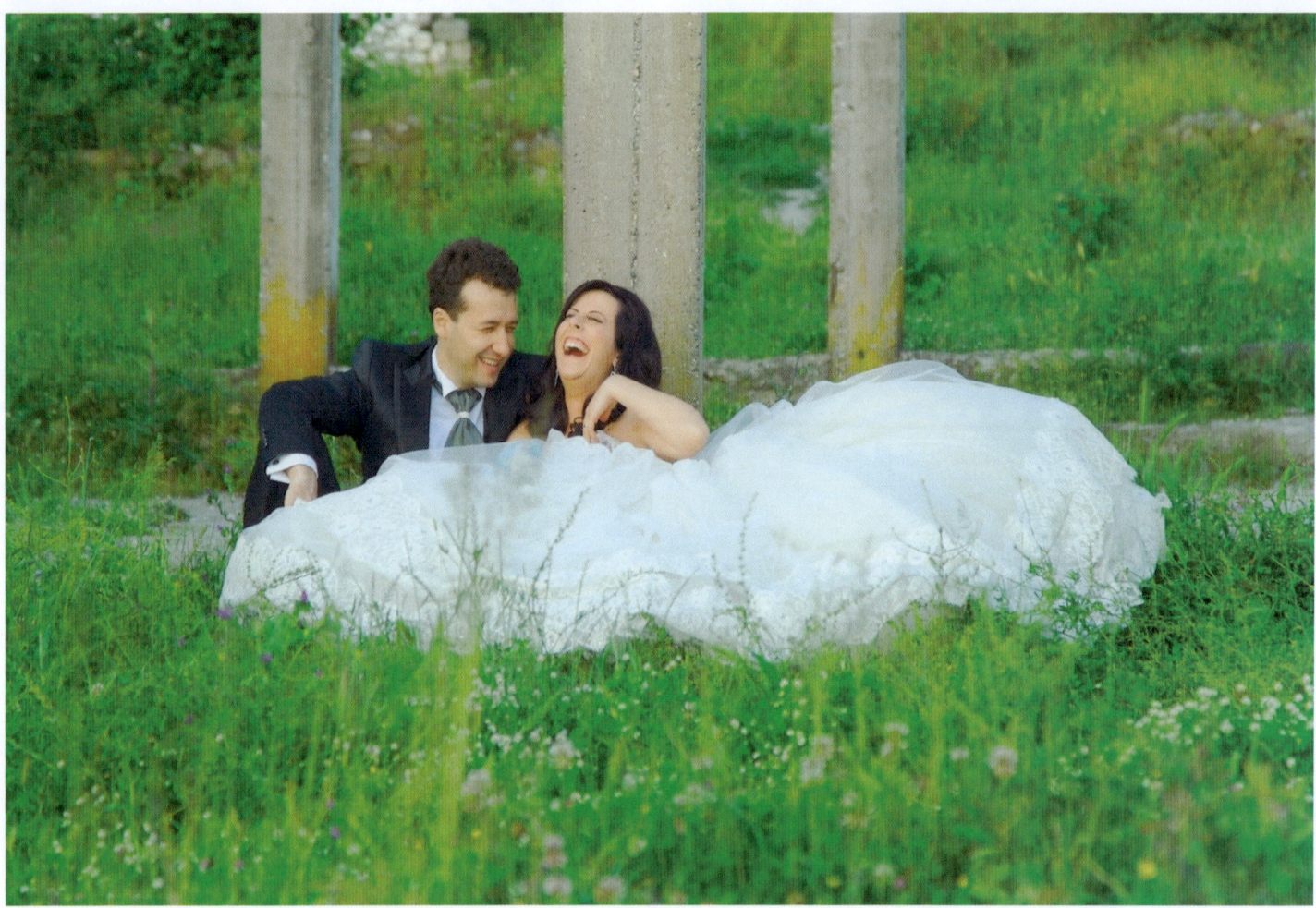

1. What day is this for the couple?

2. Why do you think they are laughing?

3. Where are they?

4. Describe a wedding you were in or attended.

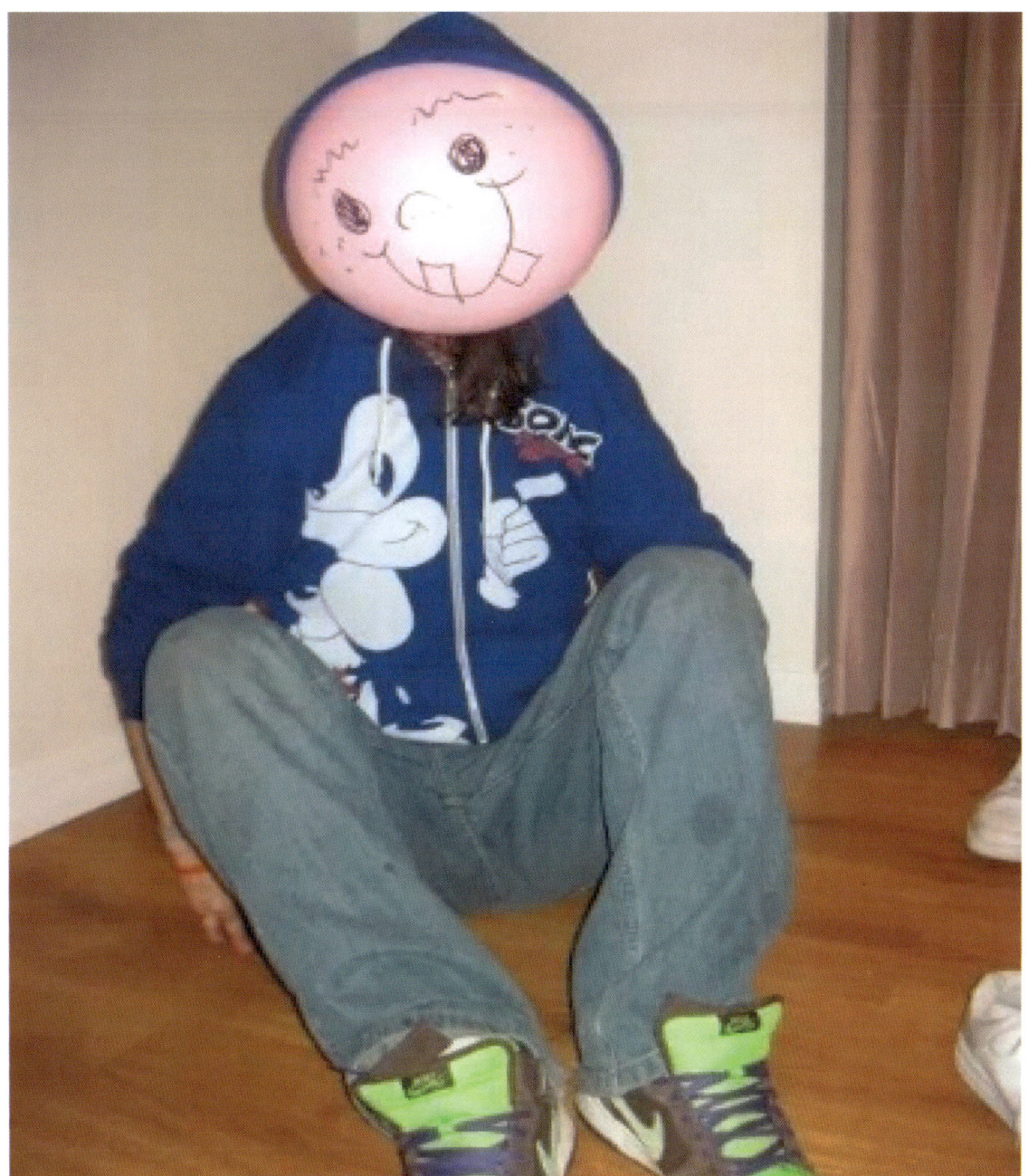

1. Describe the photograph.

2. What is bizarre about this person?

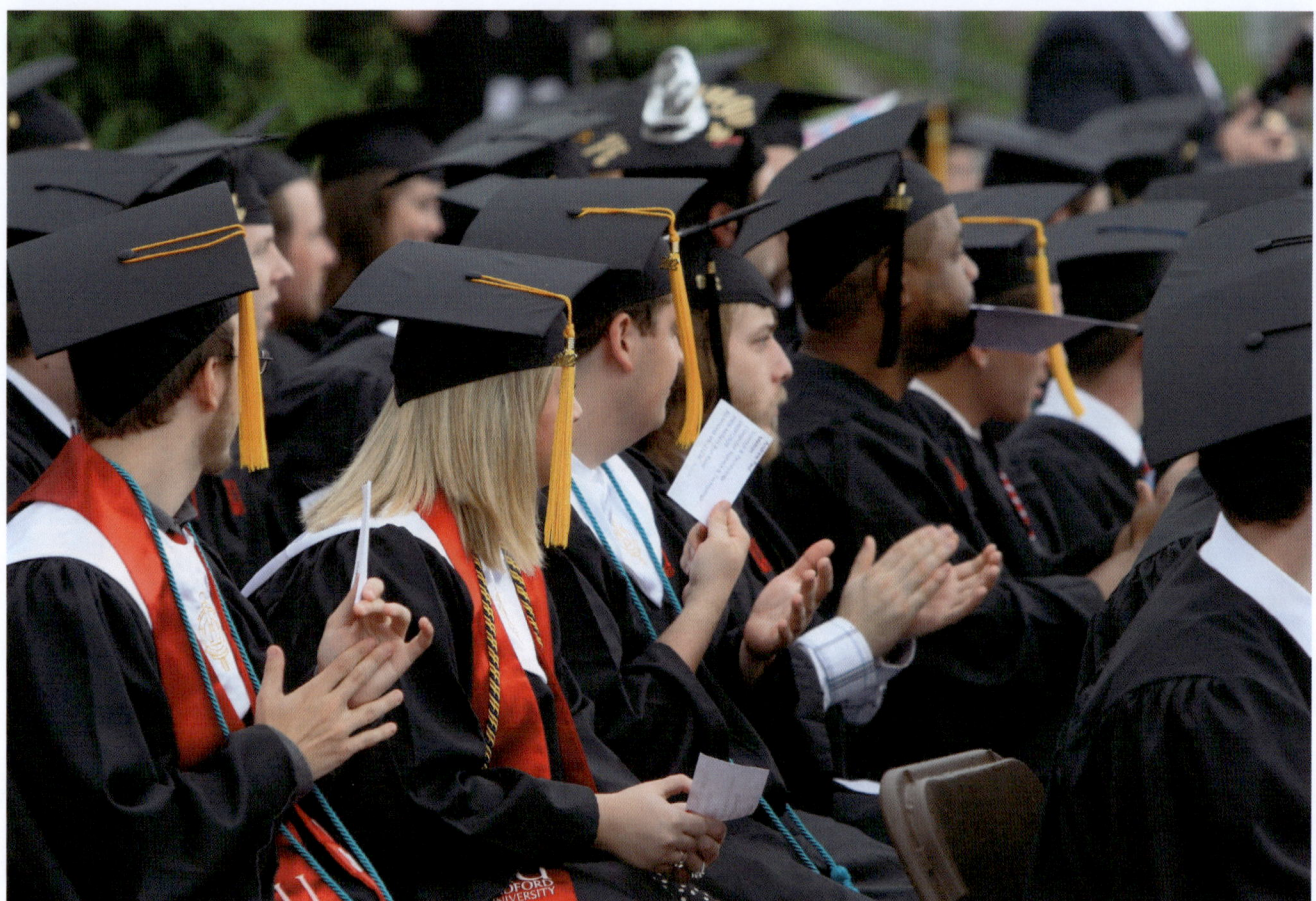

cxxi

1.   Describe the outfits in the photograph?

2.   What event is this?

3.   What graduations have you attended?

4.   What do they do with their hats sometimes at the end of the ceremony?

5.   Describe what the ceremony means.

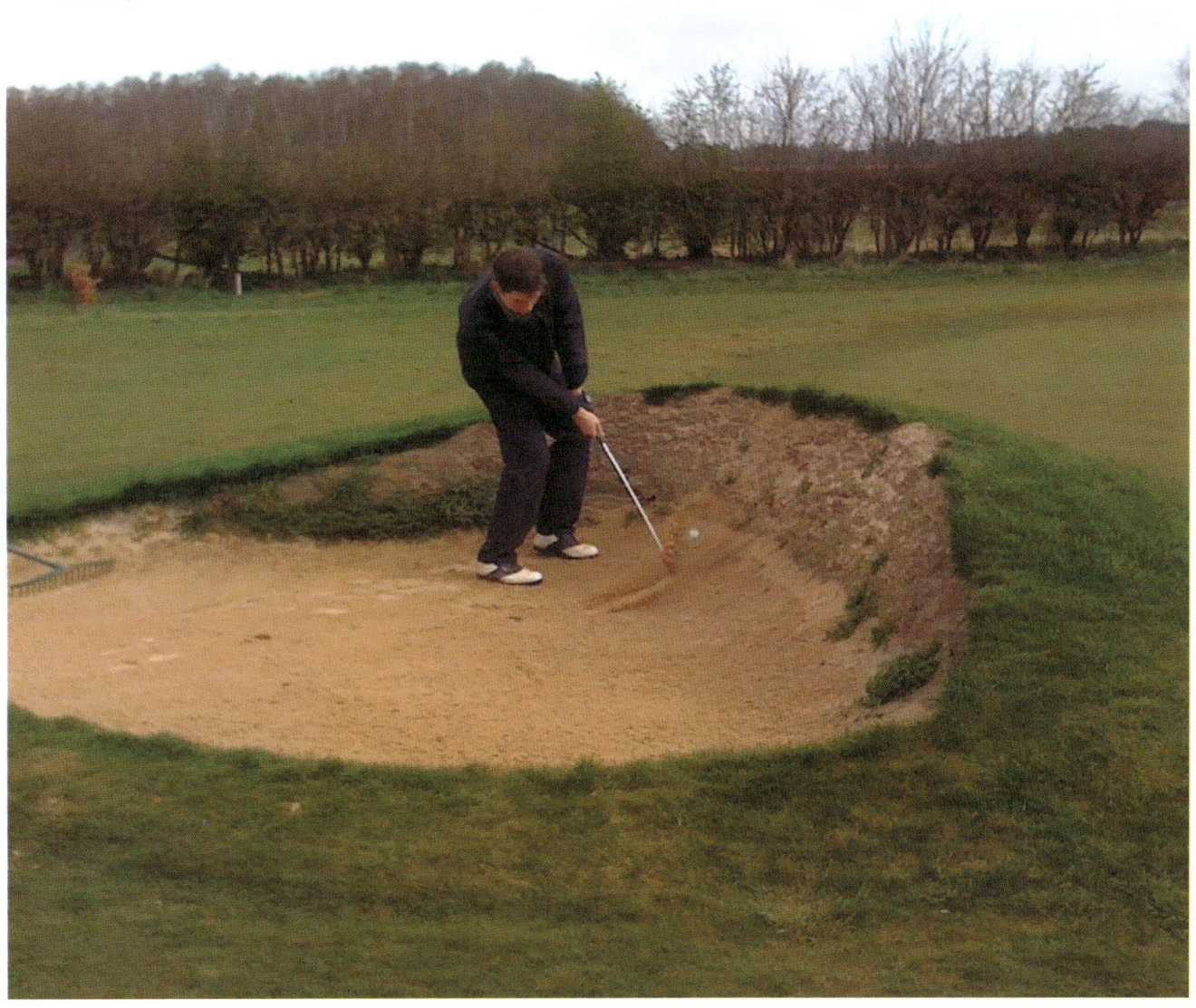

cxxii

1. What game is this?

2. Explain the objective and rules of golf.

3. Describe what the man in the photo is trying to do.

4. Did he want to hit the ball in the sand pit?

5. What is your favorite sport?

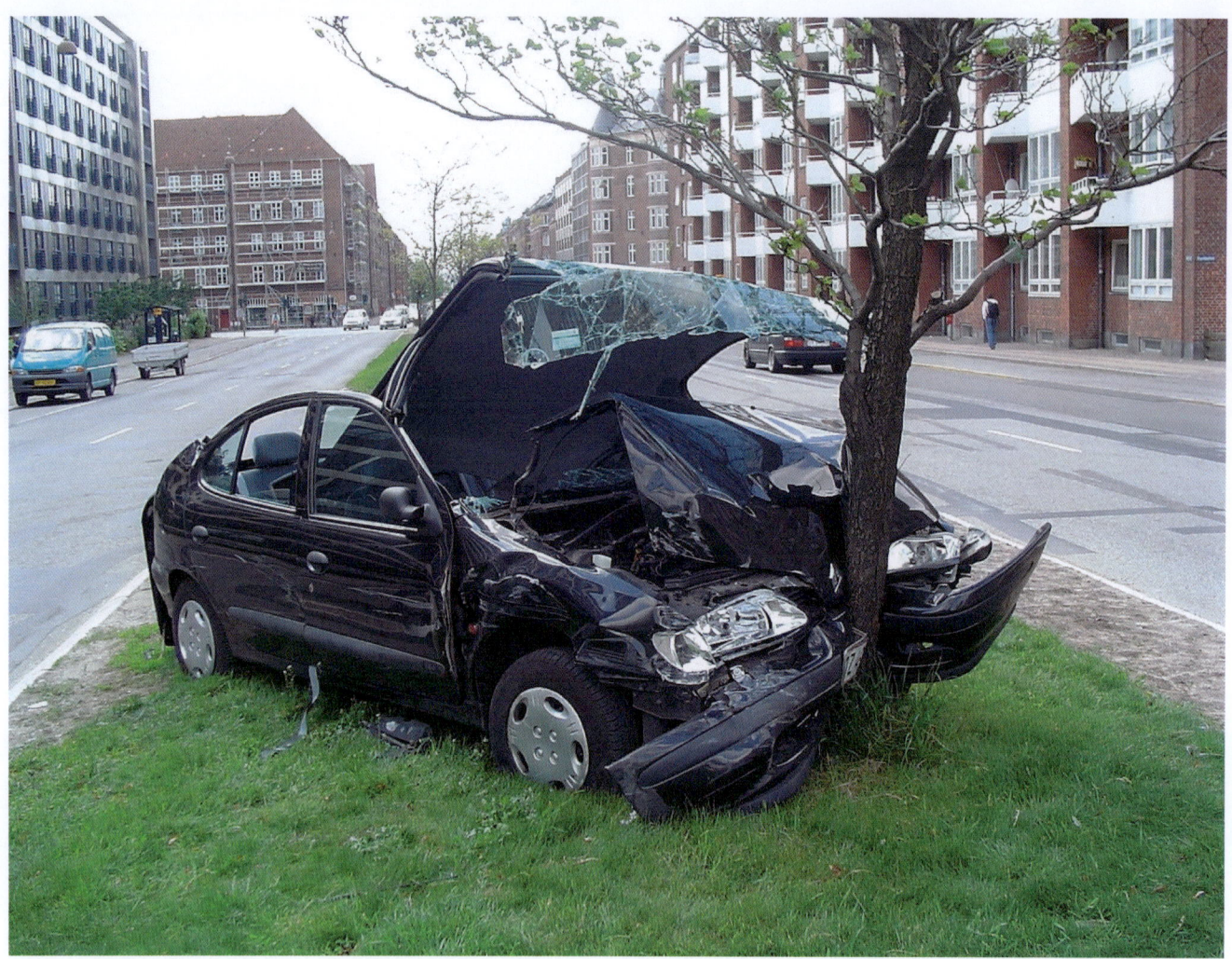

1.   What happened?

2.   What parts of the car are damaged?

3.   How would you describe the tree?

4.   Why do you think the driver went off of the road?

5.   Do you think the driver was hurt? Why? Why not?

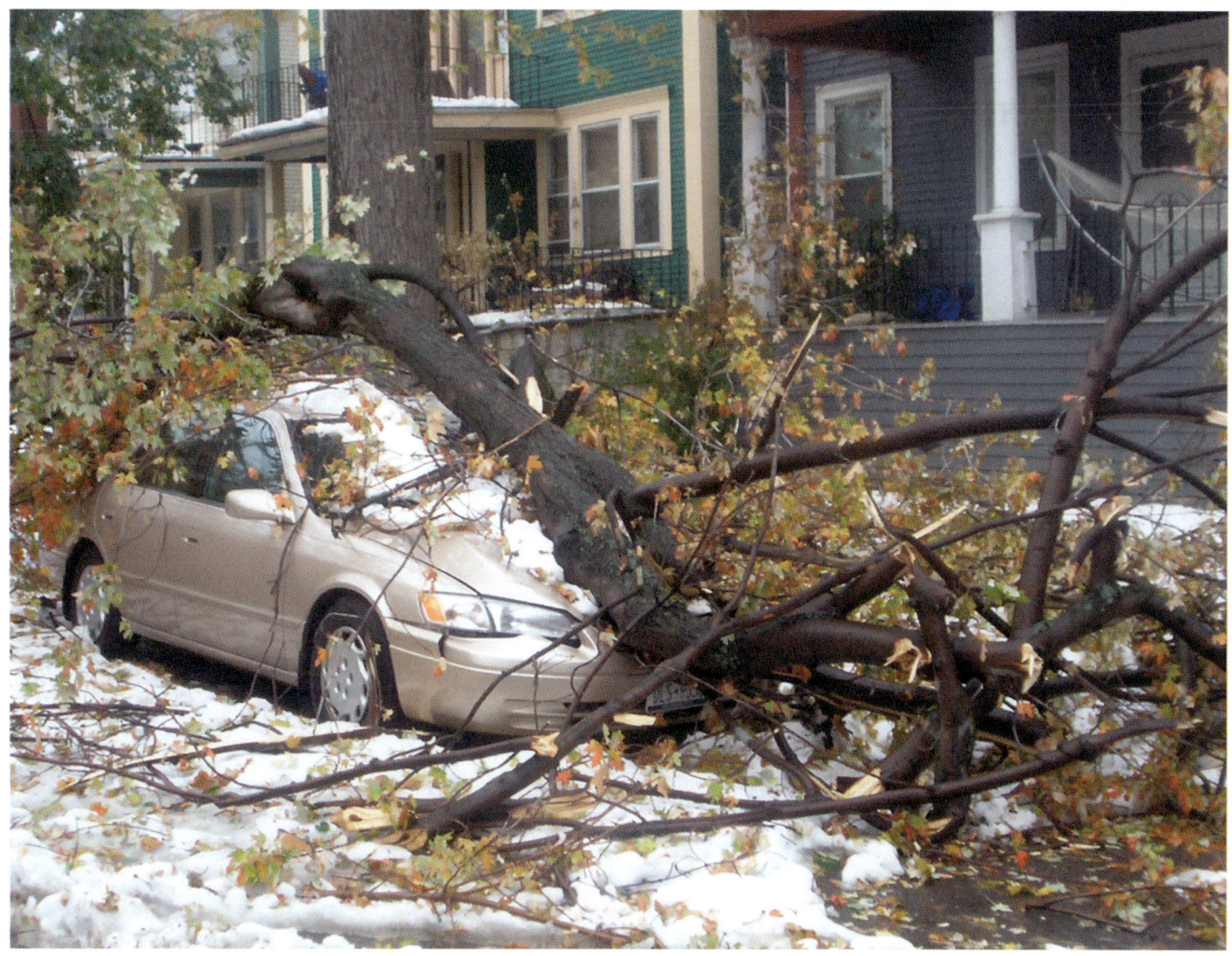

cxxiv

1.   What happened?

2.   What do you think caused the tree to fall?

3.   Do you think anyone was hurt? Why? Why not?

4.   What will the owner of the tree need to do?

5.   Pretend you own the car and call your insurance. What will you say?

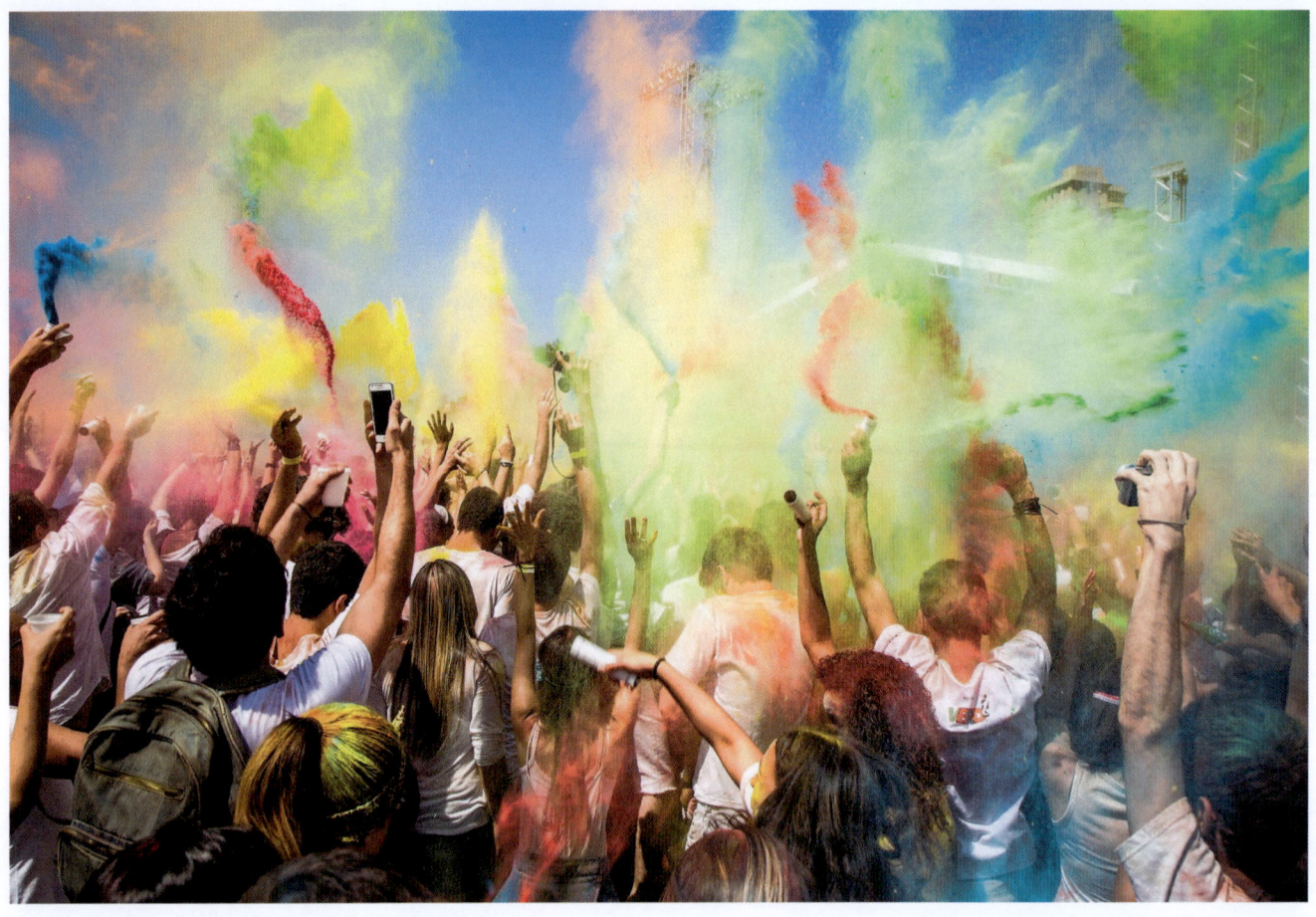

cxxv

1. Describe the photograph.

2. Name all the colors in the photo.

3. What do you think is going on?

4. This is the Hindi festival of love and color called Holi. Anybody is fair game to douse with colors. Would you like to participate?

5. Have you ever seen anything like this?

i   Source: NASA, CC-BY, via:
     http://commons.wikimedia.org/wiki/Category:NGC_6946#mediaviewer/File:NGC_6946.jpg
ii   Source: Author's photo via: Mike Anderson.

iii Source: Author's photo: via Mike Anderson.
iv   Source: Author's photo via: Mike Anderson.

v   Source: Author's photo via: Mike Anderson.

vi   Source: Melancholie, CC-BY , via: http://commons.wikimedia.org/wiki/File:Sea_Turtle.jpg

vii Source: Author's photo via: Diane Schneider.

viii Source: Forest Wanderer, CC-BY, via: http://commons.wikimedia.org/wiki/File:Cascade-falls_-_Virginia_-_ForestWander.jpg

ix   Source: Yathin S Krishnappa , CC-BY, via:
     http://commons.wikimedia.org/wiki/File:Chamaeleo_namaquensis_(Walvis_Bay).jpg

x   Source: PJ , CC-BY, via:
xi   Source: Ciudadanodemexico, CC-BY, via: http://commons.wikimedia.org/wiki/File:Shih_Tzu.jpg
xii Source: Elma, CC-BY, via: http://commons.wikimedia.org/wiki/File:Gullfiskur.jpg
xiii Source: Micha Luki, CC-BY, via: http://commons.wikimedia.org/wiki/File:Small_flip-flops.jpg.

xiv Source: Warburg, CC-BY, via: http://commons.wikimedia.org/wiki/File:BE_Kursaal_chandelier.jpg
xv   Source: Evan-Amos, CC-BY, via: http://commons.wikimedia.org/wiki/File:Tivo-remote.jpg
xvi Source: Lelê Breveglieri, CC-BY, via: http://commons.wikimedia.org/wiki/File:Ozotic_nail_polish.jpg
xvii Source: Takk, CC-BY, via: http://commons.wikimedia.org/wiki/File:Rainbow_in_Budapest.jpg
xviii Source: Kropsoq, CC-BY, via: http://commons.wikimedia.org/wiki/File:Gunte_002.jpg
xix Source: Javier8aflores , CC-BY, via:
     http://commons.wikimedia.org/wiki/File:Alejandra_Salazar_cabeza_de_huevo.jpg
xx   Source: Warren Layton, CC-BY, via: http://commons.wikimedia.org/wiki/File:Black_KitchenAid_Mixer.jpg.
xxi Source: Evan-Amos, CC-BY, via: http://commons.wikimedia.org/wiki/File:Smores-Microwave.jpg
xxii Source: ShakataGaNai, , CC-BY, via:
     http://commons.wikimedia.org/wiki/Category:Canoes#mediaviewer/File:BWCA_Canoe_Outing_-_001.jpg

xxiii Source: Evan-Amos, CC-BY, via: http://commons.wikimedia.org/wiki/File:Lipton-mug-tea.jpg.
xxiv Source : Evan-Amos, CC-BY, via: http://commons.wikimedia.org/wiki/File:Cherry-Tomatoes-in-Pack.jpg.
xxv Source: Evan-Amos, CC-BY, via: http://commons.wikimedia.org/wiki/File:Standard-lock-key.jpg.
xxvi Source: Evan-Amos, CC-BY, via:http://commons.wikimedia.org/wiki/File:Claw-hammer.jpg.
xxvii Source: Evan-Amos, CC-BY, via: http://commons.wikimedia.org/wiki/File:Honeywell-Pentax-Spotmatic.jpg.
xxviii Source: Kevin Law, CC-BY, via: http://commons.wikimedia.org/wiki/Lamb#mediaviewer/File:Sheep%2C_Stodmarsh_6.jpg.
xxix Source: Evan-Amos, CC-BY, via: http://commons.wikimedia.org/wiki/File:Duct-tape.jpg.

xxx Source: Evan-Amos, CC-BY, via: http://commons.wikimedia.org/wiki/File:Red-Pepper.jpg.
xxxi Source: Evan-Amos, CC-BY, via: http://commons.wikimedia.org/wiki/File:Crayola-Markers.jpg.

xxxii Source: Evan-Amos, CC-BY, via http://commons.wikimedia.org/wiki/File:McD-Quarter-Pounder-wCheese.jpg.
xxxiii Source Evan-Amos, CC-BY, via: http://commons.wikimedia.org/wiki/File:Tool-hacksaw.jpg.

xxxiv Source Evan-Amos, CC-By, via: http://commons.wikimedia.org/wiki/File:Brown-Mens-Boots.jpg
xxxv Source: Brian0918, CC-BY, via: http://commons.wikimedia.org/wiki/File:Conch_shell_2.jpg.
xxxvi Source: Magnus Manske, CC-BY, via:
     http://commons.wikimedia.org/wiki/Category:Buses#mediaviewer/File:ARRIVABUS_WRIGHTBUS_GEMINI_II_RO
     UTE_79D_AT_LIVERPOOL_ONE_BUS_STATION_JULY_2013_%289313900931%29.jpg
xxxvii Source: Poca a Poca, CC-BY, via: http://commons.wikimedia.org/wiki/Template:Potd/2014-06#mediaviewer/File:Pit
     %C3%B3n_de_la_India_%28Python_molurus%29%2C_Zoo_de_Ciudad_Ho_Chi_Minh%2C_Vietnam%2C_2013-08-

14%2C_DD_08.JPG

xxxviii Source: MK2010, CC-BY, via: http://commons.wikimedia.org/wiki/File:Cloth_Suitcase.jpg

xxxix Source: Shrolok, CC-BY, via: http://commons.wikimedia.org/wiki/File:Rockingchair.JPG.

xl Source: Hellbus, CC-BY, via: http://commons.wikimedia.org/wiki/Template:Potd/2014-06#mediaviewer/File:Pit%C3%B3n_de_la_India_%28Python_molurus%29%2C_Zoo_de_Ciudad_Ho_Chi_Minh%2C_Vietnam%2C_2013-08-14%2C_DD_08.JPG

xli Source: Aine D, CC-BY, via: http://commons.wikimedia.org/wiki/File:Tunisian_crochet_pillow.jpg.

xlii Source: Masa, CC-BY, via: http://commons.wikimedia.org/wiki/Fan#mediaviewer/File:Kawasaki-Electric_Fan.jpg.

xliii Source: author's photo via: Kenneth Lauria.

xliv Source: author's photo via: Kenneth Lauria

xlv Source: author's photo via: Kenneth Lauria

xlvi Source: author's photo via: Kenneth Lauria

xlvii Source: author's photo via: Kenneth Lauria

xlviii Source: author's photo via: Kenneth Lauria

xlix Source: author's photo via: Kenneth Lauria

l Source: author's photo via: Kenneth Lauria

li Source: author's photo via: Kenneth Lauria

lii Source: lolaire, CC-BY, via, http://commons.wikimedia.org/wiki/File:Statue_of_Liberty.jpg.

liii Source: Tobi87, CC-BY, via: http://commons.wikimedia.org/wiki/Grand_Canyon#mediaviewer/File:Grand_Canyon_NP-Arizona-USA.jpg/

liv Source: Leonardo Da Vinci, CC-B& via: http://commons.wikimedia.org/wiki/Mona_Lisa#mediaviewer/File:Mona_Lisa%2C_by_Leonardo_da_Vinci%2C_from_C2RMF_retouched.jpg

lv Source: Benh, CC-BY, Via: http://commons.wikimedia.org/wiki/Eiffel_Tower#mediaviewer/File:Tour_Eiffel_Wikimedia_Commons.jpg.

lvi Source: Mabdalla, CC-BY, via: http://en.wikipedia.org/wiki/File:EgyptianPyramidsandSphinx2006.jpg.

lvii Source: **Talmoryair** CC-BY, via: http://commons.wikimedia.org/wiki/Sistine_Chapel_ceiling#mediaviewer/File:Lightmatter_Sistine_Chapel_ceiling2.jpg

lviii Source: Bernard Gagnon, CC-BY, via: http://commons.wikimedia.org/wiki/Stonehenge#mediaviewer/File:Stonehenge_02.jpg

lix Source: Craig Nagy,

lx Source: Cele4, CC-BY, via: http://commons.wikimedia.org/wiki/Great_Wall_of_China#mediaviewer/File:GreatWall6.jpg. http://commons.wikimedia.org/wiki/Mount_Rushmore_National_Memorial#mediaviewer/File:Mtrushmore3cele4.jpg.

lxi Source: Yann, CC-BY, via: http://commons.wikimedia.org/wiki/Taj_Mahal#mediaviewer/File:Taj_Mahal%2C_Agra%2C_India_edit2.jpg.

lxii Source: Clindberg, CC-BY, via: http://commons.wikimedia.org/wiki/Washington_Monument#mediaviewer/File:WashMonument_WhiteHouse.jpg.

lxiii Source: Boris Dzhingarov, CC-BY, via: http://commons.wikimedia.org/wiki/File:Niagra_Falls_-_Waterfalls_(9856066165).jpg.

lxiv Source: Eddau, CC-BY, via: http://commons.wikimedia.org/wiki/File:Reacher_Assistive_Technology_a1.jpg/

lxv Source: Gramody, CC-BY via: http://commons.wikimedia.org/wiki/File:Grab_bar.jpg.

lxvi Source: Ceil, CC-BY, via: http://commons.wikimedia.org/wiki/File:Douchestoel.JPG.

lxvii Source: C-Tek permission granted to publish via: http://www.c-tec.co.uk/products/conventionalcall.htm.

lxviii Source: Center for Disease Control, CC_BY, via: http://commons.wikimedia.org/wiki/File:Chair_and_walker_easier_to_sit_down_and_rise.jpg/

lxix Source" Author's photo via: Kenneth Lauria.

lxx Source: Author's photo via: Kenneth Lauria.

lxxi Source: Author's photo via: Kenneth Lauria.

lxxii Source: Author's photo via: Kenneth Lauria.

lxxiii Source: CDC, CC-BY, via: http://phil.cdc.gov/phil/details.asp

lxxiv Source: Rennett Stowe, CC-BY, via : http://commons.wikimedia.org/wiki/File:Start_of_a_Horse_Race_(3431708779).jpg

lxxv Source: Rennett Stowe, CC-BY, via
 :http://commons.wikimedia.org/wiki/File:Thoroughbred_Horse_Race_(3445325751).jpg
lxxviSource: Rennett Stowe, CC-BY, via: http://commons.wikimedia.org/wiki/File:Strait_Of_Dover_Queens2012.jpg
lxxvii

lxxviiiSource: **Justin Black** , CC-BY, via: http://commons.wikimedia.org/wiki/File:Jaguar_kills_caiman_1.jpg

lxxixSource: **Justin Black** , CC-BY, via: http://commons.wikimedia.org/wiki/File:Jaguar_kills_caiman_2.jpg

lxxxSource: **Justin Black** , CC-BY, via: http://commons.wikimedia.org/wiki/File:Jaguar_kills_caiman_4.jpg

lxxxiSource: Florian Fuchs, CC-BY, via:
 http://commons.wikimedia.org/wiki/File:Sprengung_Aussichtsturm_Pyramidenkogel-002.jpg

lxxxiiSource: Florian Fuchs, CC-BY, via:
 http://commons.wikimedia.org/wiki/File:Sprengung_Aussichtsturm_Pyramidenkogel-004.jpg

lxxxiii Source: CDC, CC-BY, via: http://phil.cdc.gov/phil/details.asp
lxxxiv Source: CDC, CC-BY, via: http://phil.cdc.gov/phil/details.asp
lxxxv Source: CDC, CC-BY, via: http://phil.cdc.gov/phil/details.asp
lxxxvi Source:CDC, CC-BY, via: http://phil.cdc.gov/phil/details.asp
lxxxvii Source: CDC, CC-BY, via: http://phil.cdc.gov/phil/details.asp.
lxxxviii Source: CDC, CC-BY, via http://phil.cdc.gov/phil/details.asp.
lxxxix Source: CDC, CC-BY, via: ttp://phil.cdc.gov/phil/details.asp.
xc   Source: Mybec, CC-BY, via: http://commons.wikimedia.org/wiki/File:Aintree_Mansion.JPG.
xci Source: LostDogPhoto, CC-BY, via: http://commons.wikimedia.org/wiki/File:Carson_mansion.jpg.
xcii Source: Tod Carpenter, CC-BY, via:
 http://commons.wikimedia.org/wiki/File:Modern_home_on_Lookout_Mountain,_2007.jpg.

xciii Source: Daderot, CC-BY, via: http://commons.wikimedia.org/wiki/File:Log_Cabin_(University_of_Pittsburgh)_-
 IMG_0799.jpg.
xciv Source: agnosticpreacherskid, CC-BY, via:http://commons.wikimedia.org/wiki/File:1417_-
 _1419_Q_Street,_N.W..JPG.
xcv Source: Muffingg, CC-BY, via: http://commons.wikimedia.org/wiki/File:Mobile_Home.JPG.
xcvi Source: ikkoskinen, CC-BY, via: http://commons.wikimedia.org/wiki/File:Lovell_Beach_House_03.jpg.
xcvii Source: Provelt CC-BY, via: http://commons.wikimedia.org/wiki/File:Cabo-San-Lucas-Playa-Solmar.jpg.
xcviii Source: SGT9nJGl, CC_BY, via: http://commons.wikimedia.org/wiki/File:Harvey_Bennett_Ranch_House.jpg.
xcix Source: Provelt, CC-BY, via: http://commons.wikimedia.org/wiki/File:Dairy_House_Farm_-_geograph.org.uk_-
 _523924.jpg.
c   Source: King of Hearts, CC-BY, via: http://commons.wikimedia.org/wiki/Template:Potd/2014-
 02#mediaviewer/File:Athene_cunicularia_-near_Goiania%2C_Goias%2C_Brazil-8_edit.jpg
ci   Source: Gorthac, CC-BY, via: http://commons.wikimedia.org/wiki/File:Butters_Ruiz.JPG
cii Source: Archaeodontosaurus CC-BY, via:http://commons.wikimedia.org/wiki/Template:Potd/2014-
 08#mediaviewer/File:Tabanus_sudeticus_MHNT_Portrait.jpg.
ciii Source: Liez, CC-BY, via: http://commons.wikimedia.org/wiki/Template:Potd/2014-
 08#mediaviewer/File:Meriones_unguiculatus_-_Wilhelma.jpg.
civ Source: U.S. Marine Corps, CC-BY, via: http://commons.wikimedia.org/wiki/Template:Potd/2014-
 08#mediaviewer/File:Aircraft_Rescue_Firefighting_training.jpg.
cv   Source: CDC, CC-BY, via http://phil.cdc.gov/phil/details.asp.
cvi Source: Author's photo via: Kenneth Lauria..
cvii Source: piotr ilowiecki, CC-BY via: http://commons.wikimedia.org/wiki/File:Fire_busker_Mardi_Gras_1984.jpg.
cviiiSource: Douglas J. McLaughlin , CC-BY, via:
 http://commons.wikimedia.org/wiki/File:Taktshang_cropped.jpg#mediaviewer/File:Taktshang.jpg
cix Source Howie Luvzus, CC-BY, via: http://commons.wikimedia.org/wiki/File:Pink_Mardi_Gras.jpg.

cx   Source: Jonathan Billinger, CC-BY, via: http://commons.wikimedia.org/wiki/File:Treehouse_and_Menhir_-
 geograph.org.uk-_371035.jpg.

cxi Source: 山脉, CC-BY, via: http://commons.wikimedia.org/wiki/File:Fire_Dragon_dance.jpg.

cxii Source: CDC,. CC-BY, via: http://phil.cdc.gov/phil/details.asp

cxiii Source: Anton Croos CC-BY, via: http://commons.wikimedia.org/wiki/File:Newborn_of_Lesser_short-nosed_fruit_bat.JPG

cxivSource: Chuck129, CC-BY, via: http://commons.wikimedia.org/wiki/File:Crazy_Father_Rob_Keighron.jpg.

cxv Source: Author's photo, via: Jenn Harrison.

cxvi Source: BotMultichillT, CC-BY, via: http://commons.wikimedia.org/wiki/Explosion#mediaviewer/File:US_Navy_020712-N-5471P-010_EOD_teams_detonate_expired_ordnance_in_the_Kuwaiti_desert.jpg.

cxvii Source: Dave Gatley, CC-BY, via: http://commons.wikimedia.org/wiki/File:FEMA_-_116_-_Photograph_by_Dave_Gatley_taken_on_09-17-1999_in_North_Carolina.jpg..

cxviii Source: CDC, CC-BY, via: http://phil.cdc.gov/phil/details.asp.

cxix Source: Mathius, CC-BY, via: http://commons.wikimedia.org/wiki/File:Hilarious_(5815469354).jpg.

cxx Source: Author's photo, via: Kevin Lauria.

cxxi Source: Author's photo, via: Mike Anderson.

cxxii Source: Phil Hawksworth, CC-BY, via: http://commons.wikimedia.org/wiki/File:Golf_bunker.jpg.

cxxiii Source: Thue, CC-BY, via: http://commons.wikimedia.org/wiki/Car_crash#mediaviewer/File:Car_crash_1.jpg.

cxxiv Source: DragonFire, CC-BY, via: http://commons.wikimedia.org/wiki/File:Buffalo_snow_storm14.jpg.

cxxv Source: Gianluca Ramalho Misiti, CC-BY, via: http://commons.wikimedia.org/wiki/File:Sem_t%C3%ADtulo_holi_festival_colours_2013.jpg.

Printed in Great Britain
by Amazon